LOOK GREAT SLEEVELESS

THE ULTIMATE WORKOUT GUIDE TO AWESOME ARMS, SULTRY SHOULDERS AND A BEAUTIFUL BUST

BRAD SCHOENFELD, CSCS, CPT

Foreword by
MINNA LESSIG
Ms. Fitness USA

Prentice
Hall Press

Library of Congress Cataloging-in-Publication Data

Schoenfeld, Brad
   Look great sleeveless : the ultimate workout guide to awesome arms, sultry shoulders and a beautiful bust / Brad Schoenfeld ; foreword by Minna Lessig.
     p. cm.
   ISBN 0-7352-0304-0 (pbk.)
   1. Bodybuilding for women.   2. Exercise for women.   I. Title.

GV546.6.W64 S35 2001
646.7'5'02—dc21   2001036820

Acquisitions Editor: *Ellen Schneid Coleman*
Production Editor: *Mariann Hutlak*
Interior Design/Page Layout: *Dimitra Coroneos*

Not all exercises or diets are suitable for everyone. Before you begin this program, you should have permission from your doctor to participate in vigorous exercise and change of diet. If you feel discomfort or pain when you exercise, do not continue. The instructions and advice presented are in no way intended as a substitute for medical counseling. The author and publisher disclaim any liability or loss in connection with the exercise and advice provided herein.

Printed in the United States of America

10 9 8 7 6 5 4 3 2

ISBN 0-7352-0304-0

ATTENTION: CORPORATIONS AND SCHOOLS

Prentice Hall books are available at quantity discounts with bulk purchase for educational, business, or sales promotional use. For information, please write to: Prentice Hall, Special Sales, 240 Frisch Court, Paramus, NJ 07652. Please supply: title of book, ISBN, quantity, how the book will be used, date needed.

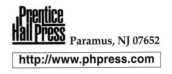 Paramus, NJ 07652

http://www.phpress.com

OTHER GREAT FITNESS PRODUCTS FROM BRAD SCHOENFELD

Books

➡ *Sculpting Her Body Perfect* (Human Kinetics, 1999)

➡ *Look Great Naked* (Prentice Hall Press, 2001)

Videos

➡ *Look Great Naked Abs*

➡ *Look Great Naked Thighs*

➡ *Look Great Naked Butt*

Be sure to check out the Look Great Naked Website at:

www.lookgreatnaked.com

CONTENTS

FOREWORD

When Brad asked me to write the foreword for *Look Great Sleeveless,* the first thing I did was make a muscle. After the quick check and reassurance of still having Popeye biceps, I decided I was representative enough of looking great sleeveless. How shallow—if it were true! Actually, the first thing I did was drop my mouth wide open to say, "Wow!" I was flattered, to say the least, and excited to promote a book so well written on weight-training the upper body.

Technique is a key element in the physical component of changing your physique. Understanding how to correctly position your body and to move it most efficiently decreases risk of injury and maximizes results. What you put into your workout is what you get out of your workout. Learning the correct technique of any exercise is a part of what I call *intelligent training,* a gateway toward increasing body awareness.

Brad has explained how to train your arms so thoroughly that this book is an educational tool not only for the consumer, but also for personal trainers and fitness teachers. You've got quality in your hands—a "Mini Me" version of Brad—that you can take to the gym for guidance through your workouts. The information is the same you would get from a top-notch fitness expert who really knows what he or she is doing, but more importantly, who really *loves* what he or she is doing.

Brad loves what he does. His knowledge of how the body moves and how to weight-train the body jumps out at you from every page. I love this! Passion, that is . . . and since Brad didn't ask me to make a muscle before asking me to endorse his book, let me share some of my own with you.

You bought this book for many reasons, some of which you already know and many of which you will uncover in time. Whatever your goal for your physical body, you have the potential to achieve it. Just listen to your heart's song, always dancing with it in life, and your dreams will unfold easily. The truth of your dreams is as real as the love in your heart, for they are outward reflections of the beauty you behold inside. Stay on that inner journey uncovering all that you can about yourself, and the rest falls easily into place.

So while you're at the gym going through the exercises in this book, talk with your body in the language of love and feel gratitude for this wonderful tool Brad has given you, and for all that you are putting into the equation. The result, of course, is looking great sleeveless, and also a delightful feeling with yourself! Your dreams are future realities. Enjoy the journey.

Health, happiness, wisdom, and love in you,

Minna Lessig
Ms. Fitness USA

ACKNOWLEDGMENTS

➡ To super-agent Bob Silverstein, for finding the proper home for this project. I couldn't have found a better agent and friend!

➡ To Debora Yost, for seeing the potential in this book and allocating the necessary resources to make it a success.

➡ To the entire Prentice Hall staff, for being so friendly and helpful.

➡ To my parents, for your continual support.

➡ To all my clients at the Personal Training Center for Women, past and present, for helping me perfect the High-Energy Fitness system and furthering my quest for self-actualization.

➡ To all the trainers who have worked at the Personal Training Center for Women, past and present, for helping me make a positive impact on the lives of many.

➡ To Clarissa Chueire, Michelle Gabriele, Kim Cardone, Cindy Goldmintz, Linda Speranza and Lisa DeGiacomo, for enduring all of those poses and making the photo shoot run so smoothly.

➡ To Joe Weider, for helping to bring fitness into the mainstream and expanding my knowledge in the early years.

➡ To the numerous professors of nutrition and exercise science who, through your teachings and writings, have furthered my knowledge in a complex field.

➡ To Minna Lessig, for your help and inspiration. I'm greatly appreciative.

➡ To Tina Jo Orban, Theresa Hessler, Karen Hulse, Cynthia Hill, Nicole Rollolazo, Jen Hendershott, Nancy Georges, Susan Balson, Connie Garner, Tatiana Anderson and Tanja Baumann, for your endorsement of this book. You are true fitness professionals!

➡ To Christina Young—the best publicist in the business. Your expertise has been invaluable in getting my message out.

INTRODUCTION

Flip through the pages of any fashion magazine and you'll notice something missing: sleeves! Slinky tube tops, sultry strapless gowns . . . virtually all the top designers are creating apparel that show off a woman's flex appeal. Without question, the sleeveless look is in and women, in turn, are becoming more and more desirous of a lean, toned upper body. While in the past women have always been concerned about their hips and thighs, over the past few years the upper body has increasingly moved to center stage.

Alas, the great majority of women still are dissatisfied with the way they look sleeveless. They shy away from the latest fashions simply because their chests, shoulders and arms aren't up to the task. As a personal trainer, hardly a day goes by that I don't hear laments such as, "How can I get rid of my bat wings?" (drooping arms), or, "Is there anything I can do to keep my breasts from succumbing to the forces of gravity?" Fortunately, the answer to these questions is a resounding "Yes!" Almost every woman has the ability to improve the appearance of her upper body and to look great sleeveless—provided she takes the proper approach. By employing the right mix of exercise and nutrition, any woman can have a great physique—regardless of her present shape.

In this, the second of my "Look Great" series of books, I present to you a customized upper body program based on my High-Energy Fitness™ system of training—a supercharged method of exercise that simultaneously tones your muscles while reducing body fat. *Bodysculpting* is at the core of my system. Simply stated, bodysculpting is a method of strength training that creates a toned, shapely physique—as opposed to *bodybuilding,* which focuses more on building big, bulky muscles. Think of each trouble zone as a mound of clay. You are the sculptor—the bodysculptor—and can mold these areas any way you choose. You can add a little here, subtract a little there—do whatever you wish to create the look that you desire. Whether you want to build up, slim down, tighten or tone, you are in control of your own physical destiny. If you put in the effort, results are guaranteed.

Better yet, the High-Energy Fitness™ program also is very time efficient. If you're like most women, you are constantly juggling your agenda, trying to fit a myriad of things into a limited amount of time. Job constraints, running a household, raising children—the chores are never-ending. With all these responsibilities, you certainly can't afford to spend several hours a day in the gym. The truth is, you don't need to. Each trouble zone requires only about fifteen minutes of training time per session. As you will see, it is the *quality* of training, not the *quantity* of training, that builds a terrific physique. In the case of exercise, less is more. Considering the minimal time commitment of my program, you can't use the excuse that it's impossible to fit a workout into your busy schedule.

Here is an overview of what will be covered:

➠ **Chapter One** provides an overview of what it takes to look great sleeveless. You'll find out the realities of body fat, why spot reduction doesn't work, the truth about bulking up and much, much more.

➠ **Chapter Two** relates strategies to help you stay motivated in your quest for achieving a better body. The biggest reason that women fail in their fitness endeavors is a lack of dedication. You'll learn specific ways to get into the right frame of mind, set attainable goals, transfer results through visualization and more.

➠ **Chapter Three** outlines the protocols for the targeted bodysculpting program. No stone is left unturned. Sets, reps, intensity—they're all covered in great detail.

➠ **Chapter Four** delves into the art of exercise performance. As the saying goes, it's not merely what you do, it's how you do it. Here you'll learn how to execute the routine so that results are optimized.

➠ **Chapters Five, Six, Seven and Eight** describe targeted training programs of the shoulders, chest, triceps and biceps, respectively. You'll learn basic muscular anatomy supported by diagrams that illustrate each muscle. Exercises are broken down into "groups" that target specific areas of your body. A total of 60 different exercises are described in explicit detail. Accompanying the exercise descriptions are photos demonstrating correct performance.

➠ **Chapter Nine** discusses the fat-burning benefits of cardiovascular exercise. Aerobics complement the targeted bodysculpting workouts, accelerating your ability to get lean and hard. But there's a lot more to aerobics than simply jumping on the bike or treadmill. All the basics are covered: frequency, duration and intensity. An overview of different cardiovascular modalities is provided, discussing the pros and cons of each.

➠ **Chapter Ten** details a complete nutritional regimen to reduce body fat and fuel your body. Proper nutrition is vital to achieving a lean, toned physique. Don't think that you can simply exercise your way to a great body—it won't happen. Nutrition is at least as important as exercise in the quest for aesthetic perfection. Many nutritional inaccuracies and untruths are debunked. There are no gimmicks here; only scientifically based concepts that have been proven to work.

➠ **Chapter Eleven** details expert tips for achieving lasting weight management. These tips are at the cutting edge of nutrition. By incorporating them into your dietary regimen, you'll turn your body into a fat-burning machine, allowing it to operate at peak efficiency.

➠ **Chapter Twelve** explains how to get your body into top shape for a specific event. It's a one-week program that's guaranteed to have you looking your very best!

➠ ***Chapter Thirteen*** contains a collection of healthy recipes contributed by some of the top fitness models in the world. These are the favorite recipes of women who make their living by keeping their bodies in top shape. You'll see that eating healthy doesn't have to be boring. Whether it's breakfast, lunch, dinner or snacks, you'll find recipes that make your mouth water.

In sum, you'll find all the information that you need to sculpt your upper body to perfection on the pages that follow; the only thing you need to do is put in the effort. With dedication and persistence, you'll be well on your way to looking great in any sleeveless outfit. And who knows, maybe one day you'll be able to grace the cover of a fashion magazine.

THE BARE ESSENTIALS

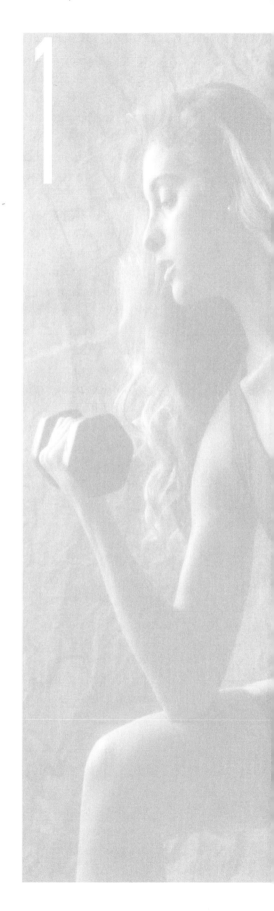

Upper Body Blues ...

With the prevalence of sleeveless outfits, you'd think that every woman would be working to attain a lean, mean upper bod, right? Wrong!

The sad fact is, many women still focus exclusively on training the "trouble zones" at the expense of their upper body musculature. Clinging to the misguided theory that targeted exercise selectively reduces fat, they'll perform endless sets of floor exercises in hopes of magically melting away their problem areas. Or worse, they'll buy the latest fat-zapping gizmo from a late-night infomercial, duped into believing that a fancy piece of machinery is the answer to a buffed physique.

Unfortunately, spot reduction is a myth—a physiologic impossibility. Despite the inflated claims made by some unscrupulous hucksters, individual exercises can't slim down a specific area of your body. It's sad but true; no matter how often or intensely you perform a particular movement, the site-specific effects on lipolysis (fat burning) are virtually nonexistent.

In order to appreciate why spot reduction doesn't work, it is necessary to understand the way in which fat is synthesized. When calories are consumed in abundance, your body converts the excess nutrients into fat-based compounds called *triglycerides,* which are then stored in cells called *adipocytes* (fat cells). Adipocytes are pliable storehouses that either shrink or expand to accommodate fatty deposits. They are present in virtually every part of the body. There is a direct correlation between the size of adipocytes and obesity: the larger your adipocytes, the fatter you appear.

When you exercise, triglycerides are broken back down into fatty acids, which are then transported via the blood to be used in target tissues for energy. Because fatty acids must travel through the circulatory system—a time-consuming process—it is just as efficient for your body to utilize fat from one area as another. In other words, the proximity of fat cells to the working muscles is completely irrelevant from an energy standpoint. Since the body can't preferentially recruit fat from a particular area, it simply draws from adipocytes in all regions of the body including the face, trunk and extremities. Hence, trying to spot reduce fat is, in reality, just an exercise in futility.

So does this mean that targeting specific body parts is superfluous? Certainly not! When performed correctly, targeted exercises help to develop lean muscle. Muscle in turn helps to build a strong, supporting "infrastructure" that prevents an area from sagging. Even with a surrounding layer of body fat, flabby areas appear firmer, remaining shapely and symmetrical. And when all the fat is finally stripped away, you're left with nothing but pleasing muscle tone.

By no means, however, should training be limited to the problem areas. Even if you don't care about the appearance of your upper body (which would be hard to understand), it's still essential to take a holistic approach to exercise. The reason has to do with the metabolic effects of muscle. For each pound of muscle in your body, you burn up to an additional 50 calories a day. Better yet, these calories are burned on a continual basis, even when you're lying on the couch watching your favorite TV program. While 50 calories might not sound like much on the surface, consider that by gaining a mere five pounds of lean muscle (which, if you're a beginner, can be accomplished in a matter of months), you'll burn an additional 1,750 calories a week. Assuming you keep food consumption constant, this will result in a net loss of about 1 pound every two weeks. That's 25 pounds of fat in just a year's time!

Accordingly, those who train only their problem areas are completely missing the boat; half of your muscle resides in the upper body and, by ignoring this fact, you're losing out on half of your body's fat-burning potential. The evidence is clear: Training your shoulders, chest and arms actually helps to reduce the flab in your butt and thighs—or, for that matter, any other area of the body where fat is stored.

I Want to Look Great Sleeveless!

Having conducted thousands of fitness assessments over the years, I can state unequivocally that the great majority of women train their upper body for aesthetic reasons; pure and simple, they want to look great sleeveless. And it's no wonder. From Hollywood starlets to elite socialites to conservative businesswomen, shoulder-baring garments are literally everywhere. And with so many styles from which to choose, there's a sleeveless outfit to suit almost any occasion.

Nowhere is sleeveless more in vogue than in the bridal arena. I get calls on an almost daily basis from women who want to get in shape for a wedding. Brides-to-be, maids of honor, bridesmaids—they all say virtually the same thing: The hottest wedding dresses are sans sleeves. So it goes without saying: In order to look great in that "special dress," you need an upper body that's up to the task.

Fortunately, the upper body tends to respond extremely well to targeted exercise, at least in terms of visible muscular tone. Here's why: Adipocytes are regulated by receptors that control the storage and release of fat from the cell. Receptors can be likened to doorways; they provide a means for allowing fat into or out of adipocytes. There are two basic types of fat receptors: *alpha* receptors and *beta* receptors. Taking the doorway analogy a step further, alpha receptors are the "entrances" that allow fat into adipocytes for long-term storage while beta receptors are the "exits" that let fat out of adipocytes to be burned for energy.

How does all this relate to muscle tone? Well, it has been shown that the lower body adipocytes have a very high ratio of alpha receptors to beta receptors (as much as 6:1, by some estimates). Given a plethora of fat-hungry alpha receptors (entrances) and only a limited amount of fat-burning beta receptors (exits), the lower body tends to hoard fat and hold on to it. That's why this area always seems to be so resistant to fat loss.

On the other hand, the upper body normally has a fairly even distribution of alpha and beta receptors (approximately a 1:1 ratio). Since "entrances" are equally matched by "exits," fat can be burned about as easily as it can be stored, keeping the upper body fairly lean. And without a layer of fat to obscure definition, results will be apparent in a fairly short period of time.

Now this doesn't hold true for everyone. The storage of body fat is unique to each individual. Albeit less frequently, some women store more fat in their arms or torso than in the lower extremities. But, generally speaking, most will find it relatively easy to develop visible upper body muscle tone.

Reaping Additional Rewards

Since you're expending all of this effort to look great sleeveless, you should be happy to know that you'll derive more from your hard work than just aesthetics. While you are sculpting your shoulders, chest and arms to physical perfection, these muscles also get stronger in the process. "So what," you say, "I just want to look great sleeveless." Well, don't underestimate the importance of upper body strength. It has a tremendous impact on your capacity to carry out activities of daily living. Hauling groceries, holding your baby, moving furniture and many, many other actions are heavily dependent on the muscles of the arms and torso. If you don't have sufficient strength in this region, basic everyday tasks will become a chore and your quality of life will decline.

From a strength perspective, females are at a physiologic disadvantage. Even when adjusted for body mass, women have only about half the upper body strength of their male counterparts (this is in direct contrast to lower body strength, which is fairly equal between the sexes). Making matters worse, strength levels diminish with age. This is largely due to a loss of muscle tissue, which approaches one percent per year after the age of about 35. Little by little, muscular function deteriorates (a condition that has been termed *sarcopenia* by the medical establishment) and, by the time the average woman reaches 60, she's already lost about one-quarter of her strength—enough to significantly impair functional capacity.

Through targeted training, these factors become moot. With dedicated effort, you actually can turn back the clock and improve upper body strength. Sarcopenia is reversed and muscular function actually improves. And the best part is that results are age-independent; even women in their 80s and 90s show significant strength improvements from a regular program of exercise.

What About Genetics?

Without question, genetic factors have a major impact on your ability to shape your muscles. Unfortunately, genetics are predetermined and cannot be altered; you can't choose your parents—at least not until human cloning is perfected! Depending on the arrangement of your muscle fibers and the insertion of your muscle attachments, there will be limits as to what you physically can accomplish. That's why it's imprudent to compare yourself to other women. Only a gifted few have the ability to look like an Olympic gymnast, fitness model, or ballet dancer. If you don't possess this basic body type, all the diet and exercise in the world won't change matters.

That said, virtually everyone has the capacity to look great sleeveless. If you have the desire to transform your body, it is within your power to do so—regardless of your genetic limitations. By training hard and eating right, you can maximize your potential and conquer your weaknesses, creating a balanced, symmetrical upper body of which you can be proud.

The important point here is to be realistic. Forget about trying to achieve the body of your favorite celebrity. Rather, evaluate your own strengths and weaknesses and just concentrate on making yourself the best that you can be. Once you get into the advanced stages of training, you can sculpt your body to make the most of your God-given attributes. As you'll see, targeted upper body training can help to create the illusion of a smaller waist, bigger chest or just about anything else you can think of. There are numerous ways to highlight your assets and hide your flaws once you discover the wonderful world of bodysculpting.

But I Don't Want to Bulk Up!

Perhaps a woman's biggest fear is that she'll bulk up from lifting weights. Biceps curls and chest presses conjure up images of big, bulging muscles—not lean muscle tone.

Even in these enlightened times, many still cling to the misguided belief that curls and presses are "manly" exercises that only serve to decrease femininity.

The truth is, however, it's *extremely* difficult for a woman to develop overly large muscles. The main reason: a lack of testosterone. Testosterone is a hormone that's secreted by the testes (in males) and, to a lesser extent, the ovaries (in females). It has two main functions. First, testosterone is *androgenic* (i.e., masculinizing); it promotes male-oriented characteristics such as the growth of facial and body hair, male-pattern baldness and deepening of the voice. Second, testosterone is *anabolic* (building); through a complex process, it interacts at the cellular level with muscle tissue to increase protein synthesis—the primary stimulus for initiating muscular growth. Hence, there is a direct relationship between testosterone and muscle mass: The more testosterone you secrete, the greater your propensity to pack on muscle.

On average, women produce only about one-tenth the amount of testosterone as their male counterparts; this is nature's way of preserving "femininity." As a result, it's virtually impossible for women to add a significant amount of muscular bulk to their frame. Without an anabolic stimulus, muscle tissue simply has no impetus to hypertrophy (get bigger) and muscular growth remains modest, even at advanced levels of training.

Now this isn't to say that a woman can't put on more muscle than she might desire. After undertaking a strength-training program, it's not uncommon for a woman to complain that she's too "bulky." But if this is your fear, don't worry. Provided you train in the manner described in this book, I guarantee that you won't bulk up. As you will see, the extent to which you maximize your body's muscle mass is entirely your own decision.

The Bottom Line

I hope by now you're convinced—if you weren't already—that training your upper body isn't an option; it's a necessity. Not only will you look great in any sleeveless outfit, but you'll also become stronger and more energetic, able to carry out tasks that you previously thought impossible.

But don't expect it to be easy! In order to achieve optimal results, you must abstain from gorging on junk foods, dedicate yourself to a regimented exercise program and endure a fair amount of temporary discomfort when you are training. There will be daily challenges that are sure to test your resolve. You'll come home from work and feel too tired to work out. You'll want to stop training as your muscles begin to burn. You'll go out to dinner and be tempted by rich desserts.

Here is where your mind must be strong. You must rationalize that you are making short-term sacrifice for long-term gains. When you don't feel like training, think about how good you'll feel after your session. When you are struggling to finish a difficult set of an exercise, think about the sense of accomplishment you'll feel from conquering your pain threshold. And when you are offered a slab of chocolate cake, think about how great you'll look in a slinky dress the next time you're out on the town. Whatever your motivation to get into shape, use it to your advantage.

The good news is that, in short order, your mind and body will become conditioned to living a fitness lifestyle. The temptation for junk foods gradually subsides, your pain threshold increases and you develop a zeal for training that makes you want to get into the gym and work out. You'll be spurred on by seeing your upper body change by the month, and you'll relish in hearing others remark on your metamorphosis.

By this point you're probably wondering just how long it will take to see these amazing results. Well, you should start to notice changes within several weeks. You'll feel tighter and firmer, and your clothes will begin to fit better. Soon, others will start to notice these changes, complimenting you on your appearance. Over the next several months, your fat will slowly melt away and in its place will be lean, hard muscle tone. And before you know it, you'll have completely revamped your physique.

Excited? You should be. Now the fun begins: Read on and get ready to look great sleeveless!

STAYING THE COURSE

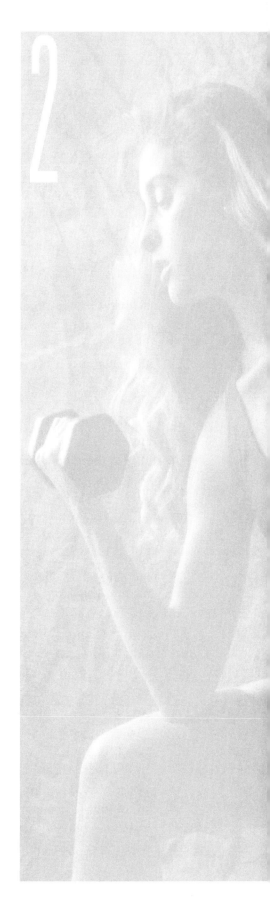

"Everyone keeps telling me how great I look ...."

While many women cannot envision ever hearing these words, it is a common statement made by those who are determined to maximize their potential. I hear these sentiments regularly from my private clients. One of my biggest joys as a personal trainer is seeing a woman's self-confidence soar to new heights because she has redefined her body.

However, in order to exact a positive change on your physique, you must be driven to succeed. It's not enough to simply want a great bod; you have to make it a priority. Almost everyone *wants* to look great sleeveless, but few have the determination to make this dream a reality.

Most women start out with the best of intentions and are brimming with enthusiasm when they begin a fitness routine. Initially, they are eager to go to the gym and are committed to attaining their best possible shape. However, within a short period of time, they begin to lose interest in working out. They start to miss workouts and stray from their nutritional regimen. Little by little, their motivation wanes. The sad fact is, after only eight weeks, more than 80 percent end up abandoning their routines altogether.

More than anything else, consistency is the key to achieving results. I can give you the perfect game plan for getting your upper body into shape, but, if you are inconsistent, you'll never maximize your potential. Once you stop an exercise regimen, all your gains gradually slip away. Your muscles atrophy, your body fat returns and you eventually appear as if you never trained at all.

Fortunately, specific actions can be taken to promote lasting compliance. By following a few basic tenets, you will be compelled to stay on the straight and narrow. Exercise is habit-forming and, once a training ritual is established, you'll feel guilty about missing a workout.

Develop a Positive Mindset

With respect to fitness, women often are their own worst enemies. They tend to be self-conscious and insecure about their bodies and perpetually see themselves as being fat and out of shape—regardless of their actual proportions. One of the distinct characteristics of anorexic women is that they are habitually obsessed with being overweight. A 5'8" runway model can look in the mirror and think she's grossly obese. This distorted sense of self-image invariably causes a woman to become despondent and give up on herself, frequently becoming self-destructive in the process.

It therefore is imperative to develop a positive body image. In spite of how you feel about your appearance, always maintain proper perspective. Never put yourself down by saying, "I'm fat," or, "I look terrible." These negative thoughts only serve to lower your self-esteem, decreasing your motivation to get into shape. Don't worry about your present condition; you are merely a work in progress. Take solace in the fact that, as long as you maintain a fitness lifestyle, every new day will bring you one step closer to achieving your ideal physique.

Get excited about the fact that you are changing your appearance. Enthusiasm and motivation go hand in hand. As the great poet Ralph Waldo Emerson once said, "Nothing great was ever achieved without enthusiasm." It's amazing how much difference a positive attitude can make in your life. Accordingly, make every effort to avoid negative people. Anyone who tries to bring you down has no place in your life. Heed the old saying: "If you hang around with dogs, you get fleas," and associate only with those who are upbeat and share your ideals. I guarantee that it will make a big difference—not only in your physique, but in your everyday life, as well.

Above all, be confident in your abilities. Strike the words "I can't" from your vocabulary. From now on, you must take the approach that you can accomplish anything you set your mind to do. And don't just think it; you must actually believe it. Believing you can do something is half the battle. To paraphrase W. Clement Stone: "Whatever your mind can conceive and believe, you can achieve."

Set Goals

Goals are essential to exercise adherence. If you have a clearly defined reason to train, you are much more likely to continue, and even look forward to, your workout. Of course, everyone has times when they simply don't feel like training. Sickness, work issues, and other crises can set back your efforts for days or even weeks. However, if you have well-defined goals that are important to you, you will be inclined to get back into your routine in relatively short order.

A goal must be both quantifiable and attainable. If these criteria are not met, the goal is non-specific and therefore not meaningful. Non-specific goals cannot be readily achieved and are apt to result in frustration. Let's discuss these criteria in greater detail:

➡ ***In order for a goal to be quantifiable, it must have measurable parameters.*** For example, losing 20 pounds in three months is a quantifiable goal. You can weigh yourself today and again in three months to see whether you have met your goal. The scale will indicate your degree of weight loss in a measurable context. Other examples of quantifiable goals include reducing your waistline by three inches in a month, dropping a dress size in six weeks, etc. Conversely, wanting to look good is *not* a quantifiable goal. This is subjective and cannot be measured by any defined standards. A "goal" like this is doomed to lead to disappointment and frustration.

➡ ***In order for a goal to be attainable, it must be realistic.*** For example, losing 20 pounds in three months is an attainable goal. Losing 90 pounds in three months is not. If a goal is not attainable, it can serve as a de-motivator. An unattainable goal can make you feel as if your fitness endeavors are pointless. It is better to set modest goals that are readily within reach. This leads to a feeling of accomplishment and spurs you on to loftier goals.

Once you have formulated your goals, break them down into short timeframes of no more than three months. By limiting the time-horizon of your goals, you are able to accomplish them in a reasonable period of time. This promotes positive feedback and buoys self-confidence. For example, losing 30 pounds might appear to be a daunting task, but losing six pounds a month for five months seems eminently more attainable. After a mere 30 days, you can relish the fact that you achieved your goal and set your sights on the next objective.

Whenever possible, create incentives to help you reach your goals. For example, if weight loss is desired, buy an expensive dress that's several sizes too small. The thought of having a beautiful dress hanging unused in your closet should be enough of an impetus to get you in the gym. Alternatively, have your husband or boyfriend agree to take you away on a romantic vacation if you drop a certain number of dress sizes. Getting others involved in your fitness efforts will provide a support network that can spur you on to greater heights. In short, think about what really motivates you and apply it to what you want to get out of your exercise program. You have to really want something in order to maintain motivation over a period of time. Without a specific goal, you will not have a reason to put in the labor necessary to achieve results. Give yourself an edge and make use of every possible motivator that is meaningful to you. It will inspire you to stay fit for life.

Once you accomplish a goal, you should immediately set a new goal that reflects your mission to work out. This will keep you focused in your efforts and allow you to maintain a high degree of motivation. Goals should be reviewed on a periodic basis to make sure that they are consistent with your present objectives. Goals will often change as you progress in your fitness endeavors, and reevaluating your position will help to ensure lasting compliance.

Visualize Success

Visualization is a technique that can be used to reinforce your goals and sustain your motivation to train. Essentially, it is an organized form of daydreaming. Many athletes use this technique to actualize their potential. A basketball player, for instance, might visualize swishing a last-second jump shot or a baseball player might visualize hitting a game-winning home run. The technique works beautifully in an exercise setting, where it has been proven to increase adherence and improve training performance.

Visualization is best practiced in a quiet environment without any distractions. It can be done either standing up or lying down. When you are ready, close your eyes and relax your muscles. Begin to think about your physique. Visualize each upper body region—your shoulders, chest and arms—and get an image of the way you want them to appear. Think of yourself in great shape, walking on the beach in a bikini, or wearing a sexy dress at a party. Make the image as clear and realistic as possible, seeing it as a movie on the back of your eyelids.

You might even want to think of a woman whose physique you admire such as a famous celebrity, fitness model or perhaps even someone who works out in your gym. Fantasize that you possess the body of your role model and carry this vision into your exercise routine. You may, for example, think of Linda Hamilton's arms or Rachel McLish's shoulders and picture them on your own body. Let your imagination be your internal source of motivation and, within reason, do not set any boundaries as to what you can accomplish.

Visualization can be enhanced through the use of photos. They say a picture is worth a thousand words. Well, it's also a great means to reinforce a specific mental image. For example, find a picture of yourself when you were happy with the way you looked and tape it to your refrigerator or put it on your dresser. Just make sure that it's in full view. Every time you see this picture, it will remind you of your potential and help to keep your image fresh in your mind.

Stay Off the Scale!

"How am I doing?" Ed Koch, the ex-mayor of New York, used to ask this question on a regular basis . . . and so does every woman who begins an exercise program. And who's to blame them? You want to make sure that all your hard work is paying off, right?

For many women, progress is measured in pounds; it all boils down to whether or not they've lost weight. Thus, the good old bathroom scale has become the preferred tool to assess the effectiveness of an exercise program. And in certain instances, the scale can be beneficial. It is convenient and easy to use; just step on the scale and you get an instantaneous readout of your weight.

Be careful, though, that you don't become a slave to the scale. Women tend to be scale-obsessed. They weigh themselves incessantly and freak out as soon as they gain a pound. In this respect, using the scale as a barometer can be deceiving and counterproductive. For instance, the scale does not account for body-fat percentage or water retention, and thus can give a false impression of actual results. Muscle is much denser than fat and consequently weighs more by volume. A golf ball, for example, weighs more than a tennis ball even though it is much smaller in overall diameter. Similarly, when you adhere to a regimented exercise program, you can actually increase your weight while decreasing your body-fat percentage. In this way, your weight is "redistributed" and you can reduce your proportions by several dress sizes.

In reality, weight is just a number and means very little in the overall scheme of things. It is much more important to be happy with your shape and like the way that your clothes fit your body. If you choose to weigh yourself, do so no more than once per week. And if you happen to gain a pound or two, take it in stride. As long as you are sticking to this program, positive change will happen—I guarantee it! In the end, defer to the mirror. Let the way you look and feel be the ultimate gauge of your progress.

PROGRAM PROTOCOLS

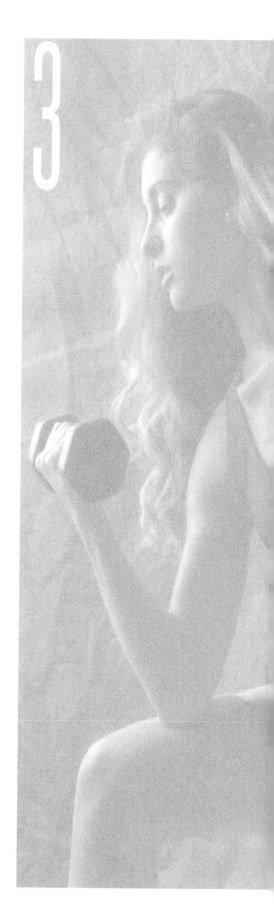

"I've tried everything but I just can't seem to get my upper body to shape up ...."

Over the years, I've heard this lament more times than I can remember. Women spend hours in the gym, riding, rowing and stepping their way to what they hope will be a better body. Unfortunately, without a proper course of action, their plight is bound to end in frustration.

There is only one way to get rid of your flab and develop a toned, shapely physique, and that's through a regimented program of exercise and nutrition. Fitness truly is the fountain of youth. It can turn back the clock and reverse the aging process, allowing you to recapture the body you once had and even improve on it. However, simply going to the gym and lifting some weights isn't enough to get the job done. The vast majority of women who undertake an exercise program never see a tangible change in their bodies. The main reason for their failure: lack of knowledge about exercise.

Exercise is a science. Just as you wouldn't attempt to overhaul a car engine without a thorough comprehension of auto mechanics, you can't expect to magically transform your physique without understanding the fundamentals of exercise. Knowledge is power! Once you've acquired the appropriate knowledge, you are in control of your body and can decide how you want it to look. You can tone, reduce, enlarge and/or shape your trouble zones to perfection. Within your own genetic potential, there is virtually no limit to what you can achieve.

Fortunately, you don't need to spend countless hours learning the rudiments of exercise physiology (although it certainly doesn't hurt). This book provides a foolproof system that takes the guesswork out of training. No stone is left unturned. Everything you need to know is laid out in a structured format, affording you the ability to concentrate on one thing: toning your upper body to perfection.

Exercises

All exercises are not alike! It is all too common for a woman to string together a series of exercises, neglecting to consider how they interact with each other. The net effect is a hodgepodge of maneuvers that have little cohesion. Ultimately, if you want to rise above the ordinary and look great sleeveless, a more scientific approach is in order.

It is a fact that certain exercises complement one another, working synergistically to produce optimal results. Others merely overlap, providing little additional utility. Unfortunately, even many seasoned fitness professionals do not fully comprehend this reality and continue to train in a haphazard fashion. This misguided approach is not only extremely inefficient, but it actually can decrease performance and compromise results.

In order to simplify the training process, exercises for the various body parts have been classified into three groups. Each group contains movements that work your muscles in a specific fashion. By choosing one exercise from each group, you'll optimally target your trouble zones without any wasted effort. All you have to do is mix and match to create a perfect routine every time. It's that easy!

There are five exercises outlined for each group for a total of 15 exercises per trouble zone: Use them all. Experiment with different combinations and strive to make each workout different from the last. This will help to counteract the adaptation process that takes place from repeatedly performing the same routine on a regular basis. When exercises are overused, your body develops a tolerance to these movements. Ultimately, you reach a training plateau and results stagnate. By employing constant variety, your muscles never can adapt to a particular exercise. Your workouts will remain a continual challenge and results will proceed at a steady rate.

Reps

Repetitions (reps, for short) are one of the least understood components of exercise. Sure, everyone knows what they are, but few understand their place in a routine. Consider the following: Several years ago, I conducted a survey of prospective clients, asking how many reps they performed in a typical set. The most common answer: "Ten." When asked why they chose to train in this rep range, the most common answer: "I don't really know!"

Clearly, the number of reps that you perform shouldn't be a mere afterthought. It is an important training variable that has a profound effect on your physique. To a great extent, it will determine the size and shape of your muscles. Let's discuss the different rep ranges and how they affect your proportions.

➠ ***High Reps:*** If you want to improve the "tone" of a muscle without substantially increasing its bulk, it is best to train in a high rep range employing between 15 to 20 reps per set. High reps target your slow-twitch muscle fibers (also called *Type I fibers*). These fibers are predominantly utilized during continuous activities sustained for long periods of time. Because of their endurance-oriented nature, slow-twitch fibers have only a limited ability to increase in size. Thus, by targeting these fibers, you'll attain a lean, toned physique with only a minimal effect on muscular mass.

➠ ***Moderate Reps:*** If you want to increase the size of a muscle, the use of moderate reps is warranted. This entails training with "heavy" weights, using between 6 to 10 reps per set. The goal here is to stimulate your fast-twitch muscle fibers— the ones that have the greatest potential for growth. These fibers (*Type II fibers*) are activated during intense, short-term activities. They are strength-oriented and therefore expand in size in order to accommodate the demands of heavy lifting. As a rule, they are the only fibers that have the ability to promote muscular bulk.

Table 3.1 summarizes the effects of training in each rep range.

TABLE 3.1
PROTOCOLS FOR REP RANGES

Rep Range	Number of Reps Per Set	Goals
High	15 to 20	Tone muscle, burn fat
Moderate	6 to 10	Build muscle

It is important to note that, depending on your goals, you can use high reps for one target zone and low reps on another. You can, for example, train your biceps with low reps to increase their size and train your shoulders with high reps to improve their definition, or vice versa. Only you can decide what rep range is better for your physique. Assess your trouble zones and select your rep range accordingly.

Regardless of the rep range you choose, it is imperative to keep your form as strict as possible. Perform each rep in a smooth, controlled manner, without allowing momentum or gravity to dictate your rep speed. If you can't finish your set within the prescribed rep range, the weight is too heavy. Resist the temptation to let your ego get in the way of results, and reduce the amount of weight to a manageable level. This will ensure complete stimulation of your target muscles and decrease the possibility of a training-related injury.

Sets

In most training programs, sets are executed in a straightforward manner. You perform a given number of reps, rest, and then repeat the process several times. However, in order to enhance definition, this program employs a technique called *giant sets*. A giant set is any set that incorporates three or more different exercises in succession. You move directly from one exercise to the next, without resting between movements. Hence, you will begin with a Group One exercise, go immediately to a Group Two exercise, and finish by performing a Group Three exercise. All told, you'll perform a total of three giant sets for each trouble zone, taking no more than 60 seconds of rest between each giant set.

During your rest intervals, you will employ a technique called *selective muscular stretching*. Selective muscular stretching is performed as follows: Upon completion of each giant set, immediately stretch the muscle being trained utilizing the stretching movements discussed below. Try to hold each stretch throughout the entire rest interval and then proceed directly to your next giant set.

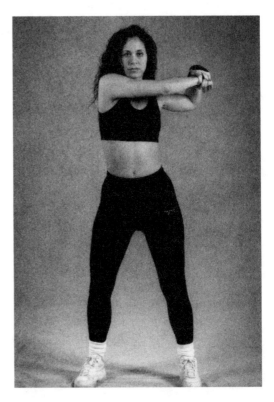

Shoulder Stretch ▶

From a standing position, grasp your right wrist with your left hand. Without turning your body, slowly pull your right arm across your torso as far as comfortably possible. Hold this position for the desired amount of time and repeat the process on the left.

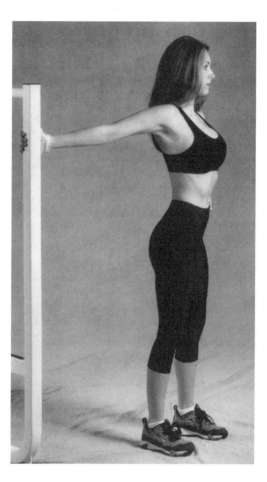

Chest Stretch ▶

From a standing position, grasp any stationary object, such as a pole or exercise machine, with your right hand. Your arm should be straight and roughly parallel with the ground. Slowly turn your body away from the object, allowing your arm to go as far behind your body as comfortably possible. Hold this position for the desired amount of time and repeat this process on the left.

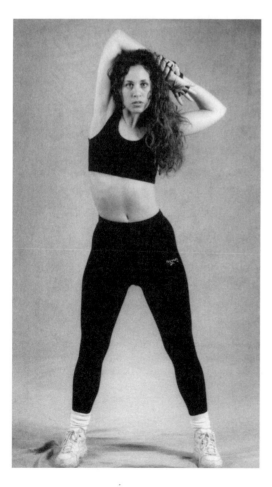

◀ Triceps Stretch

From a standing position, raise your right arm over your head. Bend your elbow so that your right hand is behind your head. With your left hand, grasp your right wrist and pull it back as far as comfortably possible, allowing your elbow to point toward the ceiling. Hold this position for the desired amount of time and repeat this process on the left.

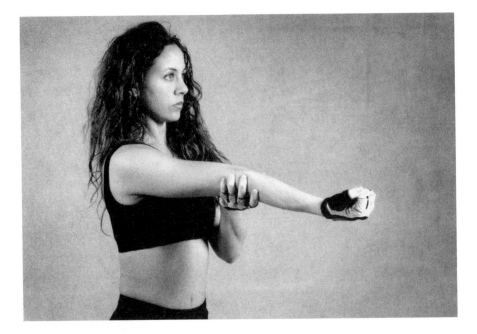

▲ **Biceps Stretch**

From a standing position, extend your right arm forward with your palm facing up. Place your left palm underneath your right elbow. Slowly straighten your right arm as much as comfortably possible, pressing your elbow down into your left hand. Hold this position for the desired amount of time and repeat this process on the left.

Selective muscular stretching helps to neutralize the effects of lactic acid by restoring blood flow to your working muscles. Lactic acid is responsible for the burning sensation that accompanies intense training and eventually impedes your ability to achieve a muscular contraction. Once it builds up, you simply cannot continue to train. By flushing this byproduct from your body, you are able to rapidly regenerate your muscular capacity, thereby improving performance.

Moreover, by expediting nutrient delivery to your musculoskeletal system, selective stretching helps to repair muscle tissue and accelerate the healing process. You experience a diminished amount of delayed-onset muscular soreness and post-workout fatigue. This results in better recuperation between workouts, allowing you to come back strong for your next training session.

Intensity

Of all the training variables, intensity is by far the most important. Simply stated, intensity is the amount of effort expended during exercise. The harder you work, the greater your intensity.

To achieve your full genetic potential, the intensity you apply must be great enough to exceed your body's work threshold—this is called the *overload principle.* By nature, the human body strives to maintain a stable state of equilibrium called *homeostasis.* If your training intensity doesn't sufficiently tax your resources, there won't be enough of a stimulus to force your body from its homeostatic state. Only by stressing your muscles beyond their physical capacity will they be compelled to produce an adaptive response and exact a change in your body.

For optimal results, you need to train with all-out intensity, taking each set to the point of momentary muscular failure. Weight training is perhaps the only activity where failure is a desired outcome. This is a strange concept for many women to grasp, and is often met with a great deal of skepticism. We live in a society where we are rewarded for our accomplishments and punished for our failures. From the time we are born, we are urged to succeed. Failure is always thought of as an unacceptable alternative. However, if you want to look your best, you need to work each muscle to its fullest extent—and that means going all out on each set.

You can't, however, expect to train with all-out intensity from the onset. Your body needs to be gradually acclimated to the effects of intense training. In order to accomplish this task, the routine is divided into three phases: conditioning, developing and sculpting. Each phase is designed to prepare your body for the succeeding phase. While time intervals are used as a yardstick for progression, don't feel that they are set in stone. Exercise is a very individualized process and you must progress at your own pace. When in doubt, it is best to err on the side of caution. Don't try to push the envelope. Most women are impatient to see results and prematurely accelerate their training intensity. Resist this temptation. If your body is not yet geared for intense exercise, you invariably will become overtrained and set back your development.

➠ **Conditioning Phase:** At the onset of training, perform each set at approximately 75% of maximum intensity. During this phase, the weights should feel somewhat heavy without causing you to struggle to complete a set. Your goal here is to condition your muscles to the rigors of training and develop the neuromuscular skills necessary for exercise performance. Focus on getting a feel for the routine, concentrating on moving smoothly between movements.

➠ **Developing Phase:** After three months, your body should be ready for a step up in intensity. At this point, intensity should be increased to about 90 percent of maximum where the last few reps of a set are a struggle to complete. Your goal here is to develop a tolerance for the discomfort associated with all-out training. Focus on working expeditiously, keeping your heart rate elevated throughout the workout.

➠ **Sculpting Phase:** After six months, your body should be fully acclimated and ready for all-out training. This means employing 100 percent intensity in your routine, going to physical failure on each set. The last repetition of a set should be extremely difficult, if not impossible, to perform. Make sure that you don't give in to the temporary physical discomfort associated with this type of training. Optimal results can only be achieved by pushing past the pain threshold and taking your body to the limit.

Table 3.2 summarizes the protocols for training intensity.

TABLE 3.2
PROTOCOLS FOR TRAINING INTENSITY

Stage	Time Frame	Level of Intensity
Beginner	Onset	75%
Intermediate	Three Months	90%
Advanced	Six Months	100%

Frequency

Contrary to popular belief, exercise doesn't build your muscles—it breaks them down. Intense training places tremendous demands on your body, resulting in a catabolism of muscle tissue, depletion of glycogen reserves, production of free-radicals and fatigue of your entire neuromuscular system. Adaptations to these aftereffects take place in the recovery period, where your body develops "muscle tone" as a way to cope with future high-intensity stresses. During recovery, your body seeks to repair, replenish and regenerate itself, becoming harder and more defined in the process.

All too often, women mistakenly subscribe to the theory that if a little bit is good, more must be better. They go to the gym and work out on a daily basis, never taking a day off. Don't fall into this trap. By shortchanging recuperation, your body will never have the chance to adequately recover from the extreme demands being placed on it. Inevitably, you will become grossly overtrained and your progress will be brought to a grinding halt. With respect to training, less can be more!

Although women have varying recuperative abilities, you never should train a muscle group on two consecutive days. As a rule, a minimum of 48 to 72 hours is necessary for adequate recovery. Become in tune with your body and know how it responds. If you are feeling fatigued or your muscles are sore, take another day off. When in doubt, it is better to rest a day and come back stronger the next.

Required Equipment

If possible, I recommend that you perform this program in a health club. A good fitness facility will have a vast array of fitness equipment available for use. In the same way that a builder uses a variety of tools to erect a house, a diversity of fitness devices are the "tools" for sculpting your body. While it may be possible for a builder to construct a house using only a hammer and saw, it obviously would be a burdensome task. The end product would be compromised, and the project would take a great deal more time than if he had a full complement of power tools at his disposal. Similarly, if your access to fitness equipment is restricted, there will be limitations on some aspects of your routine. Inevitably, this will serve to delay or restrain your progress.

With that said, for some women financial and/or logistical concerns prevent them from training in a gym. If this is your predicament, don't fret. The program is perfectly suited to be performed at home. Although you'll be slightly limited in your choice of exercises, there still are plenty of options to create a varied routine. Accordingly, where applicable, I have provided alternative home-based movements for many of the gym-based exercises. If you should opt to go it at home, you will need the following equipment:

➠ **Dumbbells:** Dumbbells are an essential component of any home gym. You probably will need a set of 2-, 3-, 5-, 8-, 10-, 12-, 15- and 20-pound dumbbells. Depending on your strength levels, additional dumbbells might be necessary.

➠ **Elastic strength bands:** Strength bands simulate cable exercise movements. Because they have a unique strength-curve, they are an excellent complement to free-weight exercises.

➠ **Bench:** Although not an absolute necessity, it is advisable to buy an adjustable weight bench. This will allow you to train at an incline, affording the ability to vary your movements and work your muscles from different angles.

Isotension

As an adjunct to your training routine, you should employ a technique called *isotension*. To many, this probably sounds like a clinical term for a new form of stress management. However, utilizing isotension can dramatically increase your muscle tone, producing the hard, defined look that women covet.

Isotension, simply stated, is the contraction of a muscle without the use of an external weight. For instance, if you flex your arm so that your biceps enlarges and hold this position, you are utilizing isotension. The same principle can be applied to any other muscle group. For instance, to harden your triceps, simply extend your arms until they are straight. Then, squeeze the triceps as forcefully as possible, feeling them getting hard and tight. Hold this contraction for about 30 seconds and then relax. After a short rest of no more than 15 seconds, repeat the process. Spend five minutes or so using the technique on your muscles after each workout; it won't take long to see results.

Other Muscle Groups

Although this program focuses on adding shape and definition to your upper body, I strongly urge you to train the rest of your body at least once per week. Your muscles function holistically, working together in an agonist/antagonist fashion. When one muscle contracts, its antagonist lengthens, creating smooth, controlled movement. Thus, neglecting areas of your body can lead to structural imbalances between muscle groups. Not only does this ruin the symmetry of your physique, but it substantially heightens the prospect of injury.

Moreover, as previously discussed, muscle tissue is metabolically active. For each pound of muscle that you add, you increase your body's fat-burning potential by 50 calories a day. If you only train select muscle groups and neglect others, a significant amount of your body's muscle-building capacity is bypassed.

For specific routines and exercises, consult my book *Sculpting Her Body Perfect* (Human Kinetics, 800-747-4457). It outlines a total-body approach to achieving your ultimate body.

Creating a Routine

As I said in the introduction, this program is not time-consuming. Each muscle group takes about 10 or 15 minutes to train, and you can work a different area each day. But although it is feasible to work out seven days a week, it is generally best to work out every other day, allowing at least 48 hours between sessions. Realize that during training you are not developing your muscles; rather, you are breaking them down. It is during rest that your body repairs muscle tissue by synthesizing protein. Ultimately, this is what produces lean muscle. Shortchanging the recuperative process can serve to diminish results.

The exact composition of your routine will depend on many things, including your goals, time schedule, recuperative abilities, training experience and other factors. One alternative is to alternate between upper and lower body workouts. If you are training on alternate days, you can perform your upper body Monday, lower body Wednesday, upper body on Friday, lower body on Sunday, etc. Since each muscle group takes about 10 to 15 minutes to complete, the whole workout should take 45 minutes or less—and you'll have several days a week when you do nothing but relax! Many other variations are possible, though, and the routine should be adapted to your specific needs.

It is also important to note that the more intensely you train, the greater the need there is to let your body regenerate. Don't overdo it! Stay in tune with your body and allow adequate rest based on your training response.

THE ART OF PERFORMANCE

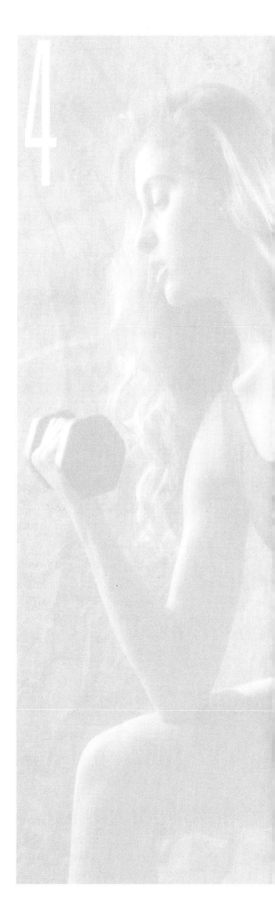

In the preceding chapter, you learned the basic protocols for targeting and toning your upper body to perfection. By following these protocols, you will be well on your way to looking great sleeveless. However, having a terrific training routine is only part of the equation. Exercise is more than just information; it also requires implementation. Without a clear grasp of proper exercise performance, you won't be able to put the protocols into practice. Ultimately, your results will be compromised and you'll fall short of reaching your potential.

It is amazing how few people actually know the correct way to exercise. Whenever I walk into a gym, I see the same training mistakes being made over and over. Sloppy form, incorrect breathing, momentum-driven repetitions—the list goes on. At best, these individuals reap only minimal rewards from their efforts; at worst, they end up suffering a debilitating injury. And being an experienced trainee doesn't ensure proper performance; many of the worst offenders have been exercising for years.

It really doesn't take much to become skilled in the fine points of exercise performance. By simply paying heed to a few key training principles, you'll be far ahead of the masses. It will take a little time before you are able to integrate these principles in a seamless fashion. But, with consistent practice, you'll soon have a firm grasp of proper lifting technique.

Perfect Form

Perfect form: Everyone wants it; few have it. Whether it's the sweet swing of a professional golfer or the effortless grace of an Olympic skater, perfect form is a thing of beauty.

In the context of weight training, perfect form involves performing an exercise so that only the target muscles are used to complete the maneuver. There are no extraneous body movements; the weight is lifted in the most efficient manner possible, allowing the muscle to directly contract in line with its fibers. There should be no hesitations and no jerky, bouncing movements—just one continuous motion, with each rep flowing smoothly into the next.

Unfortunately, most women learn how to train through trial and error. They'll watch a fitness show on cable or read a magazine and somehow believe they know how to train. Virtually no effort is made to learn exercise fundamentals. The end result can be frightening. Movements are performed in a fashion that bears little resemblance to the way they're supposed to look. And, since they don't realize that their technique is amiss, these women continually make the same mistakes time and again.

Perfect form doesn't come naturally. Even if you're athletically inclined, you can't expect to walk into a gym and breeze through your workout. The human body always tries to take the path of least resistance. It automatically attempts to lift a weight in the easiest possible fashion, not in a way that maximizes muscle tone. Thus, without a clear grasp of proper technique, your secondary muscles will take stress away from your target muscles. Ultimately, structural imbalances are created, resulting in disproportionate development of your physique. Worse, your joints become unduly stressed during exercise performance, heightening the possibility of sustaining a training-related injury.

I have furnished detailed descriptions for every exercise in this book. Make an effort to commit them to your subconscious memory, but don't simply memorize these movements; understand their function. Know the purpose of each exercise and be aware of the specific muscles that are activated in their performance. As you progress, try to gain insight into the subtleties of exercise biomechanics. The fact is, even minor adjustments in technique can make a big difference in your results.

EXPERT TIP

Always train a muscle over its full range of motion. This allows you to achieve more forceful muscular contractions. There is a direct correlation between the amount of applied force and muscular development; the greater the force, the better your development. Hence, only by working a muscle over its full range will optimal results be attained.

Remember the ABCs

The subject of rep speed has been a source of great debate among fitness professionals. At one end of the spectrum are those who advocate the use of super-slow reps. They feel that weights should be lifted at a virtual snail's pace, taking up to 15 seconds to perform a rep. On the other end of the spectrum are the speed-rep proponents. They believe in training explosively, performing reps in rapid succession. So who's right? In truth, while both of these theories have certain benefits, neither is very practical. Clearly, for the woman who wants to look great sleeveless, a middle ground is more appropriate.

With respect to rep speed, remember the ABCs of lifting—Always Be in Control. It is relatively unimportant how fast a repetition is performed, as long as the weight remains under control throughout the exercise (unless you are trying to improve speed-strength, in which case explosive movements are beneficial). Control is directly influenced by gravitational force which, in turn, is dictated by the two phases of a repetition—concentric reps and eccentric reps.

Concentric reps (sometimes called *positives*) involve lifting a weight against the force of gravity. For example, in the biceps curl (see page 107), this involves flexing your arm from a fully straightened position. During the concentric phase, you shorten the target muscle until a contraction is achieved at the top of the movement. Here, significant exertion is required to complete the lift. Because of the effort involved, a slightly faster pace is acceptable; take approximately two seconds to complete this phase.

Alternatively, eccentric reps (sometimes called *negatives*) move *with* the force of gravity. In the example of the biceps curl, this involves straightening your arm from a fully flexed position. During the eccentric phase, the muscle is lengthened and stretched at the end of the movement. Your focus here should be on resisting the pull of gravity so that momentum does not play a significant role in performance. On average, the negative phase should last twice as long as the positive, taking about four seconds to complete.

Finally, avoid the tendency to speed up as you approach the end of a set. The last few reps are always the most challenging. Not only are you fatigued, but your muscles experience the intense burn associated with lactic acid buildup. At this point, it's only natural to try to get the set over with as fast as possible. Don't give in to this temptation! Instead, become oblivious to the discomfort and maintain a steady pace. The pain is only temporary; the payoff is well worth it.

EXPERT TIP

Try to maintain a rhythm as you train. Rhythm is an essential part of exercise. It helps you establish a training groove, keeping your concentration on the task at hand. Once a pulse is established, you will settle into a comfortable training pace. As long as you are in a controlled rhythm, your rep speed will take care of itself.

Don't Hold Your Breath

What can be more natural than breathing? Breathing is the essence of life, a basic function that is innate from the time you are born. You don't need to think about taking a breath—you just do it.

Yet, during weight training, breathing becomes complicated. Rather than breathing naturally, you must inhale and exhale in sync with each repetition—a process that requires conscious thought. This often causes a woman to become discombobulated and lose focus. It's hard enough just struggling to perform an intense set with perfect form; having to remember when to breathe only serves to confuse the situation. Fortunately, within a short period of time, proper breathing becomes second nature.

You must, however, make sure to learn correct technique from the onset; once you fall into bad habits, they can be hard to break. For best results, breathing should be regimented in the following manner: Begin by taking a deep breath before commencing your set. As you initiate the concentric portion of the rep, start to exhale, expelling your breath in an even manner. By the time you contract your target muscle, all of the air should be fully released from your lungs. Then, on the eccentric portion of the movement, inhale as you return the weight to the start position, preparing yourself for the next repetition. Continue breathing in this fashion until your set is completed.

Under no circumstances should you ever hold your breath throughout a lift (a phenomenon known as the *valsava maneuver*). Doing so causes a dramatic increase in intra-abdominal blood pressure, which cuts off the blood supply to your brain. Complications such as headaches, dizziness and fainting are apt to occur. In extreme cases, you can even rupture a blood vessel or tear a retina. Needless to say, the consequences can be dire. The bottom line: Even if you breathe incorrectly, it is better than not breathing at all.

EXPERT TIP

A good way to regulate breathing patterns is to count your reps out loud. On each repetition, count in deliberate fashion: wo-one, two-oo, three-ee, etc. Make sure that you actually *say* the words; don't just mouth them. This will ensure that air passes through your vocal chords and is expelled on the contraction. As long as you continue counting, it's impossible to miss a breath! Moreover, you won't need to think about breathing properly, freeing your mind to focus on the set.

Mind in Muscle

Mind in muscle? To most, this sounds like a contradiction in terms. After all, muscle is normally associated with feats of strength, not acts of intellect. Similarly, there is a prevailing misconception that weight training is merely the action of lifting a weight from point A to point B. All too often, women think that by mindlessly performing a few sets of an exercise, they'll magically transform their physique into a work of art. Sadly, those who subscribe to this theory are doomed to fall short of their aspirations.

Contrary to popular belief, lifting weights is more than just a physical endeavor. Your mind plays an important role in the development of your physique and, in order to maximize gains, it is essential to harness your mental acuity. In fact, two women using identical exercise routines will achieve vastly different results depending on their mental approach to training. There is no doubt: If you want to look great sleeveless, it is essential to use your mind, as well as your body, during your workout.

You need to develop a mind-to-muscle connection in order to get the most out of your efforts. Simply stated, a mind-to-muscle connection is the melding of mind and muscle so that they become one. It entails visualizing the muscle you are training and feeling that muscle work throughout each repetition. Rather than thinking about where you feel a muscular stimulus, you must think about where you are *supposed* to feel the stimulus. While this concept may seem ethereal at first, in short order, its benefits will become readily apparent.

Establishing a mind-to-muscle connection is beneficial on two levels. First, it ensures that your target muscles perform the majority of work during an exercise. Otherwise, your supporting muscles and connective tissue tend to dominate the lift, diminishing your results. Second, it forces you to continually utilize proper exercise form. When you are mentally locked in to a movement, your biomechanics automatically fall into place. This not only helps to improve exercise performance, but it substantially reduces the possibility of a training-related injury.

Developing a mind-to-muscle connection requires consistent practice. From the moment you begin a set, your thoughts must be fixated on the muscle that you are training. You must be oblivious to your surroundings, with all outside distractions purged from your mind. Forget about your nail appointment, your dinner reservations or any other diversions that might arise. The only thing that matters at this point is the task at hand: sculpting your target muscles to perfection. As you train, make a concerted effort to visualize your target muscles doing the work, without assistance from supporting muscles. When you reach the contracted phase of the movement, consciously feel the squeeze in your target muscles. And, on the negative, feel your target muscle lengthening as you return to the start position. Throughout each set, make this practice a ritual. In short order, it will become habit.

Don't be discouraged if it takes longer to develop a mental link with certain muscles than with others. Generally speaking, it is easier to mentally connect with the muscles of your arms than it is with those of your torso. However, with dedication and patience, you soon will be able to connect with all the muscles in your body, paving the way to better development.

EXPERT TIP

Your mind-to-muscle connection can be enhanced through the use of a technique called *guided imagery*. Guided imagery is an extension of visualization (discussed in Chapter 2). With this technique, you visualize the way you want your muscles to look and then imagine them taking this form as you are training. For instance, when working your triceps, envision yourself with firm, defined arms, devoid of any body fat. As you perform a set of overhead triceps extensions, think of your arms becoming tighter and harder. Make the image as vivid as possible. With each repetition, see yourself getting one step closer to achieving your ultimate goal. By tapping into the power of your subconscious mind, you can take your body to new heights, turning fantasy into reality.

SULTRY SHOULDERS

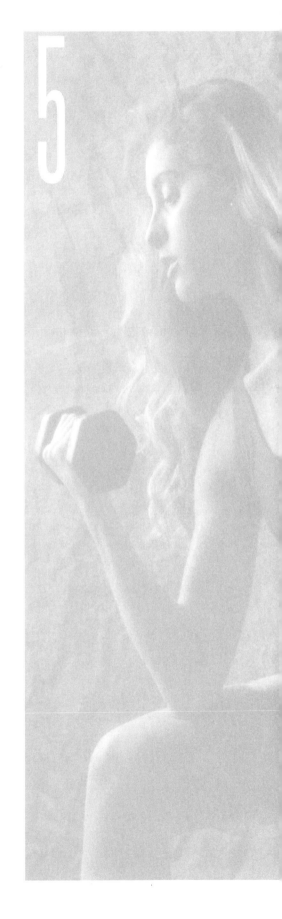

When it comes to the shoulders, women tend to be somewhat apathetic. While the chest and arms get all the glory, the shoulders are often the "forgotten child." Hence, they are usually trained as a mere after-thought, without receiving a great deal of individual attention.

Make no mistake, though, the shoulder muscles are one of the most aesthetically pleasing muscle groups. They delineate the shape of your entire body, from the outer contours of your deltoids on down. That's right, nothing does more to highlight your physique than a sultry set of shoulders.

The fashion industry is well aware of this fact. The top designers routinely insert shoulder pads into their garments. This provides instant gratification to those who lag in the shoulder area, creating an hour-glass figure without any sweat or effort. Sounds good, doesn't it?

But the problem is, you can't hide poor shoulder development when you go sleeveless; there are no shoulder pads in a tube top or tankini. It's just you and your bare essentials—a sobering thought if you don't have the necessary attributes. Yes, there's simply no getting around it; if you want to wear slinky outfits, nicely shaped shoulders are an absolute must.

To a certain extent, the length of your clavicle (collarbone) determines your shoulder-shaping ability; the longer your clavicle, the greater your potential for shoulder development. This is a genetic concern that can't be changed. Your bone structure is immutable; if it is less than ideal, you have no choice but to make do and work with what you've got.

Strength is another limiting factor in achieving optimal shoulder development. The reason is related to the function of the deltoids (delts, for short). The delts are designed to exert maximum force in movements where an object is either lifted sideward or overhead. Yet very few times in life do people ordinarily perform these kinds of tasks. Think about it. When do you ever carry something with your arms directly out at your sides? Or how frequently are you required to press an item up into the air? If you're like most women, the answer is not very often. There just aren't many activities of daily living that significantly challenge the delts and, without an impetus for remaining strong, their weight-bearing capacity progressively diminishes (the "use it or lose it" principle).

Complicating matters, the shoulder joint is the most freely mobile of all the joints in the body. It can move in almost any direction: forward, backward, up, down, sideways—the possibilities are virtually boundless. But with increased mobility comes decreased stability. In order to compensate for a large freedom of movement, the shoulder joint is loosely constructed—a fact that makes it extremely fragile and, therefore, highly susceptible to injury.

Despite these limitations, the shoulders generally respond very well to regimented exercise. Targeted training not only improves the appearance of your shoulders, but it can help to offset certain structural flaws in other areas of your body, as well. For instance, by increasing your shoulder-to-waist differential, you can develop a natural V-taper that creates the illusion of a slimmer midsection. Greater shoulder dimension also helps to even out your hips, producing more balanced and symmetrical proportions. All of the other muscle groups, no matter how perfectly developed, lose some of their impact in the absence of well-defined shoulders.

Targeted training also enhances shoulder function. While the shoulder joint is relatively feeble in the initial stages of an exercise program, it readily adapts to the rigors of training and grows strong over time. Before you know it, everyday tasks become easier to perform, leading to a better quality of life.

What's more, as the muscles and supporting connective tissue strengthen, the shoulder joint becomes increasingly more stable. This, in turn, reduces the possibility of injury—a fact that shouldn't be taken lightly. A loss of shoulder function can be debilitating, interfering with almost everything you do. Even the simplest of tasks, such as feeding yourself or getting dressed, becomes complicated if shoulder function is compromised. Worse, once the shoulder is damaged, it often is never the same afterward.

It should be noted that, in otherwise healthy individuals, the use of specific "rotator cuff exercises" is superfluous. Without question, the rotator cuff muscles (supraspinatus, infraspinatus, teres minor and subscapularis) play an essential role in stabilizing the shoulder joint. They act in concert to keep the head of the humerus (upper arm bone) in the shoulder socket. But these muscles receive both direct and indirect stimulation during most shoulder activities. The supraspinatus, for instance, receives a tremendous amount of work during the lateral raise. The infraspinatus and teres minor are highly active during reverse flyes. Thus, unless you have a specific injury or imbalance in the rotator cuff, there is no need to include isolated internal or external rotation movements in your routine (as in the so-called "flasher" exercise that mimics an exhibitionist opening and closing his raincoat).

Anatomy of the Shoulders

The shoulders comprise a variety of different muscle groups. For our purposes, however, the focus will be on the deltoids and upper trapezius. Let's take a look at the form and function of each muscle:

➠ The ***deltoid*** (delts, for short) is a triangular-shaped muscle that is comprised of three distinct "heads," each having a separate function. The anterior (frontal) deltoid flexes the shoulder joint (raises the arm in front of the body). The medial (middle) deltoid abducts the shoulder joint (raises the arm out to the side, away from the body's midline). The posterior (rear) deltoid horizontally extends the shoulder joint (brings the arm across and toward the back of the body). It is important to realize that, while the various heads can be targeted, they can't be completely isolated from one another. The deltoid functions synergistically. Depending on the movement, other heads act as stabilizers, maintaining stability in the shoulder joint.

➠ The ***trapezius*** (traps, for short) is a long, triangular muscle that runs down the entire back of the body. It originates at the base of the skull and has numerous attachments along the veterbrae, clavicle and scapula. Because of its configuration, the traps essentially operate as three different muscles and can be classified into upper, middle and lower regions. While all aspects of the traps are involved in shoulder joint movement, it's the upper traps that are most closely associated with the shoulders. The main function of this region is to elevate the scapula, shrugging the shoulders up to the neck.

Figure 5.1 provides an anatomical diagram that shows the location of the shoulder muscles.

FIGURE 5.1
Shoulder Muscles

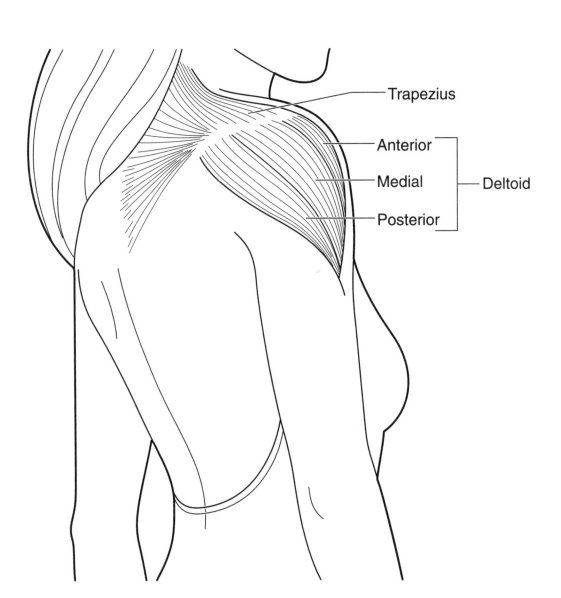

Shoulder "Dos and Don'ts"

The following points should be kept in mind during shoulder training.

➠ ***Don't*** *tense your neck during shoulder training.* Neck pain is frequently associated with shoulder training. Due to the structural interrelationship between the muscles of the shoulders and neck, it is common for a woman to reflexively tense her neck muscles as she performs shoulder movements. In many cases, a stiff neck is the aftermath.

➠ ***Do*** *consciously force the deltoids to lift the weight,* keeping the neck muscles relaxed at all times. When training the shoulders, follow the basic rule of thumb: Be intense, not tense.

➠ ***Don't*** *hyperextend your lower back during shoulder training.* In an effort to lift heavier weights, women often exaggerate the arch in their lumbar region. This provides increased leverage for completing a repetition. There are two problems here, though. First, the chest muscles are brought into the movement, taking stress away from the deltoids. Second, increased torque is placed on the lower back, heightening the potential for injury.

➠ ***Do*** *keep your lower back tight,* maintaining a normal lumbar curve at all times. Allow your abdominals and erector spinae (lower back muscles) to stabilize your torso so that no movement takes place below the shoulders.

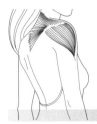

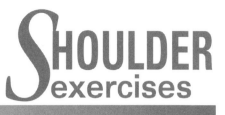

SHOULDER
exercises

Group One

Group One exercises focus on overall shoulder development, with an emphasis on the anterior (frontal) deltoid. This is accomplished by performing various types of shoulder presses. During pressing movements, the anterior delt is the primary muscle mover, with supplemental involvement from the medial and, to a lesser extent, posterior heads. In addition, the trapezius, clavicular (upper) portion of the pectorals, triceps and many other stabilizer muscles also are active to varying degrees.

Some women try to target the anterior deltoid by performing front raises. This is largely unnecessary. The front delt is worked in virtually all chest movements and generally is overdeveloped in comparison to the other two heads. Hence, unless you have an imbalance in the anterior deltoid, there is no need to perform isolated exercises for this area.

During exercise performance, make sure to avoid locking out your elbows when you reach the finish position. This only serves to increase stress on the joints while diminishing stimulation to the target muscles. Ultimately, you'll just end up with sore joints and poor muscular development. Rather, stop just short of a full lockout, keeping constant tension on the deltoids at all times.

Group 1

DUMBBELL SHOULDER PRESS (page 35)

ARNOLD PRESS (page 36)

MACHINE SHOULDER PRESS (page 37)

MILITARY PRESS (page 38)

BEHIND-THE-NECK PRESS (page 39)

34

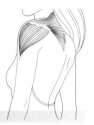

DUMBBELL SHOULDER PRESS

Begin by sitting at the edge of a flat bench. Grasp two dumbbells and bring the weights to shoulder level with your palms facing away from your body. Slowly press the dumbbells directly upward and in, allowing them to touch together over your head. Contract your deltoids and then slowly return the dumbbells along the same arc to the start position.

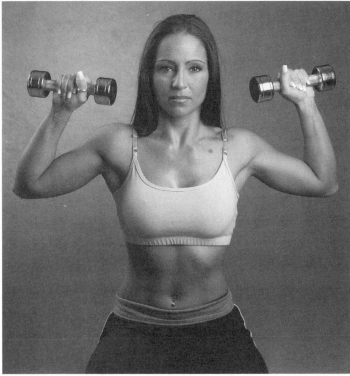

start

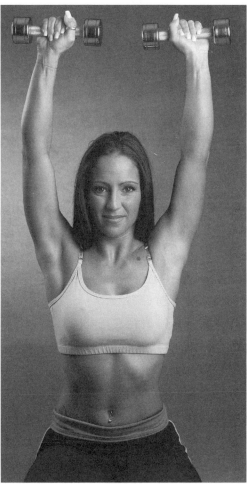

finish

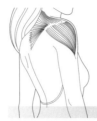

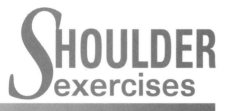

ARNOLD PRESS

Begin by sitting at the edge of a flat bench. Grasp two dumbbells and bring the weights to shoulder level with your palms facing toward your body. Press the dumbbells directly upward, simultaneously rotating your hands so that your palms face forward during the last portion of the movement. Touch the weights together over your head and then slowly return them along the same arc, rotating your hands to the start position.

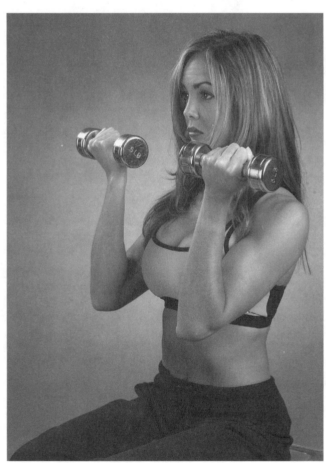

start

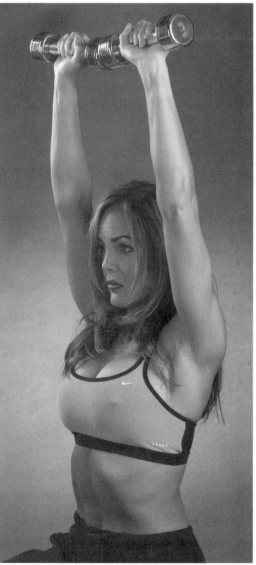

finish

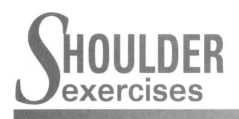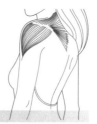

SHOULDER exercises

MACHINE SHOULDER PRESS

Begin by sitting in a shoulder press machine. Grasp the machine handles with your palms facing away from your body. Slowly press the handles directly upward and over your head, contracting your deltoids at the top of the move. Then, slowly return the handles to the start position.

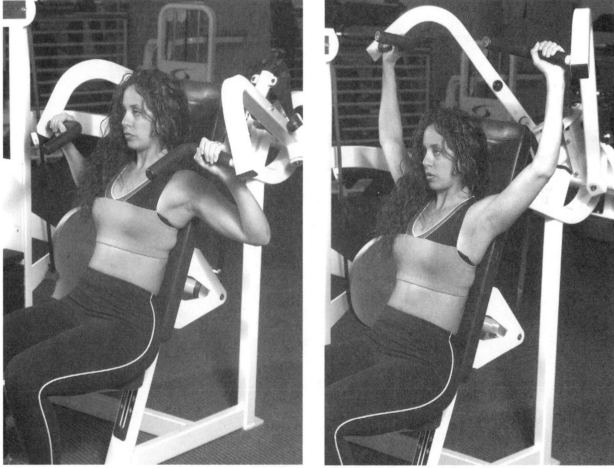

start　　　　　　　　　　　　　　　*finish*

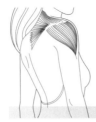
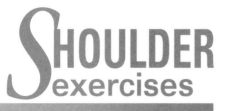
MILITARY PRESS

Begin by sitting at the edge of a flat bench. Grasp a barbell and bring it to the level of your upper chest with your palms facing away from your body. Slowly press the barbell directly upward and over your head, contracting your deltoids at the top of the move. Then, slowly return the bar along the same arc to the start position.

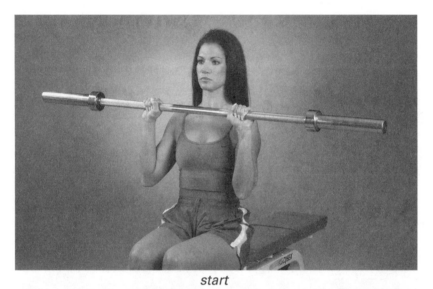

start

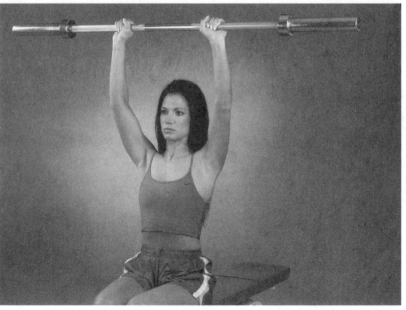

finish

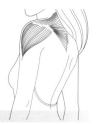

SHOULDER exercises

BEHIND-THE-NECK PRESS

Begin by sitting at the edge of a flat bench. Grasp a barbell and bring it behind your neck with your palms facing away from your body. Slowly press the barbell directly upward and over your head, contracting your deltoids at the top of the move. Then, slowly return the bar along the same arc to the start position.

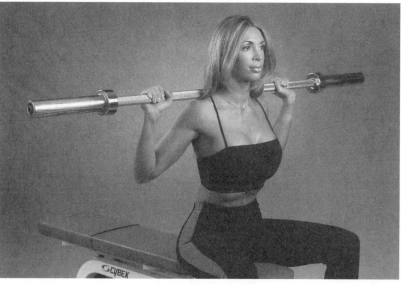

start

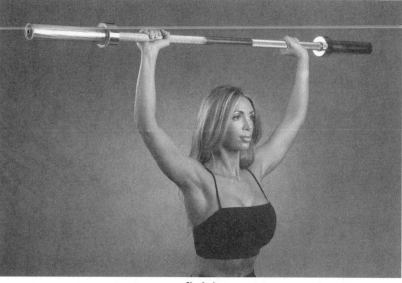

finish

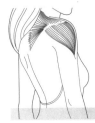

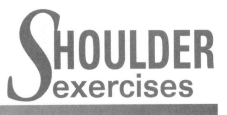

Group Two

Group Two exercises target the medial (middle) head of the deltoid. This is accomplished by performing movements that employ shoulder joint abduction (bringing your upper arm out to the side and away from the midline of your body). From an aesthetic standpoint, the medial delt is the most important of all the shoulder muscles. It is responsible for promoting shoulder width and, when properly developed, creates the illusion of a smaller waist.

Specifically, there are two basic types of abduction exercises: lateral raises and upright rows. Lateral raises are single joint movements that really focus on the medial delt. To ensure optimal stress on this aspect of the muscle, keep your elbow rigid and make sure that your pinky is higher than your thumb throughout the move (slight internal rotation). Upright rows, on the other hand, are compound movements and therefore require the activation of many different upper body muscles. However, by maintaining a shoulder-width grip and lifting directly from the shoulders (not the hands, as so often is the case), the medial delt becomes the prime mover and receives most of the stimulation.

It is important to avoid raising your upper arm beyond 90 degrees (the point where the elbow is parallel to the ground) during these moves. When abduction is combined with internal rotation, the greater tubercle of the humerus (upper arm bone) approaches the acromium (part of the shoulder blade). This tends to cause impingement of the supraspinatus tendon and long head of the biceps when the arm passes 90 degrees—a consequence that can lead to a debilitating injury. Hence, make sure to bring your arm up only until it reaches a position parallel to the ground.

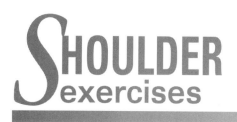

SHOULDER exercises

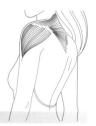

DUMBBELL LATERAL RAISE

Begin by grasping two dumbbells and allow them to hang by your hips. With a slight bend to your elbows, raise the dumbbells up and out to the sides until they reach shoulder level. At the top of the movement, the rear of the dumbbells should be slightly higher than the front. Contract your deltoids and then slowly return the weights along the same path to the start position.

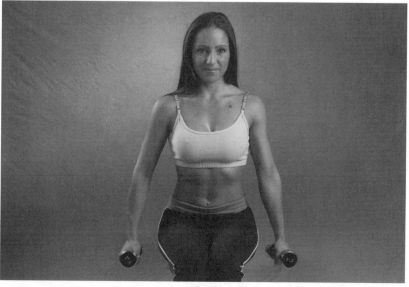

start

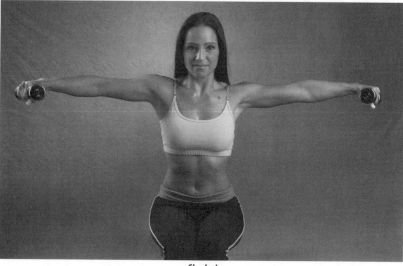

finish

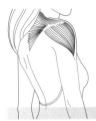

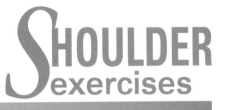

CABLE LATERAL RAISE

Begin by grasping a loop handle attached to a low pulley apparatus with your left hand and stand so that your right side is facing the pulley. With a slight bend to your elbow, raise the handle across your body, up and out to the sides until it reaches the level of your shoulder. Contract your delts at the top of the movement and then slowly return the handle to the start position. After completing the desired number of reps, repeat the process on your right side.

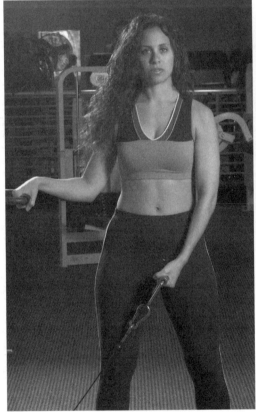

start

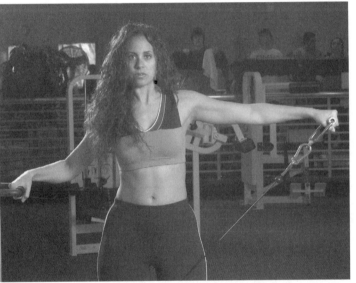

finish

For Home Use:
Attach a strength band to a stationary object and perform the move as described. ▶

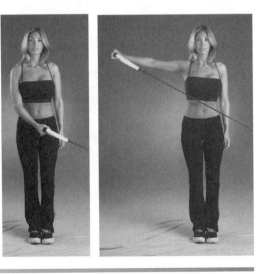

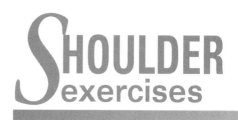

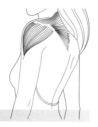

MACHINE LATERAL RAISE

Begin by sitting face-forward in a lateral raise machine. With a slight bend to your elbows, grasp the machine handles with your palms facing one another. Raise your arms up and out to the sides until they reach shoulder level. Contract your delts and then slowly return to the start position.

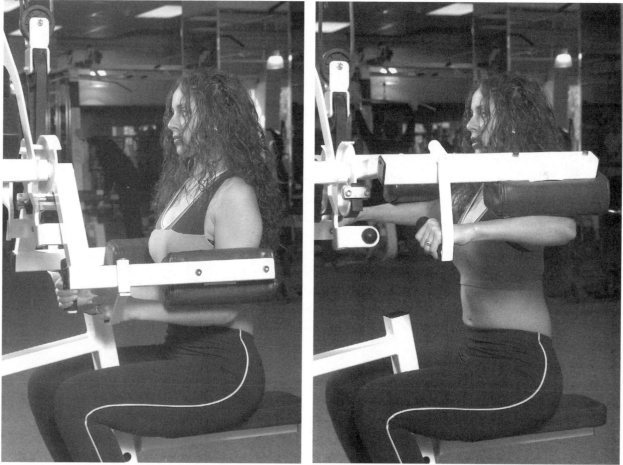

start   *finish*

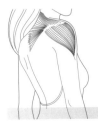

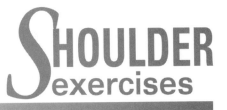

DUMBBELL UPRIGHT ROW

Begin by grasping two dumbbells. Allow your arms to hang down from your shoulders with your palms facing in toward your body. Assume a comfortable stance and keep your knees slightly bent. Keeping your elbows higher than your wrists at all times, slowly raise the dumbbells upward along the line of your body until your upper arms approach shoulder level. Contract your delts and then slowly lower the dumbbells along the same path to the start position.

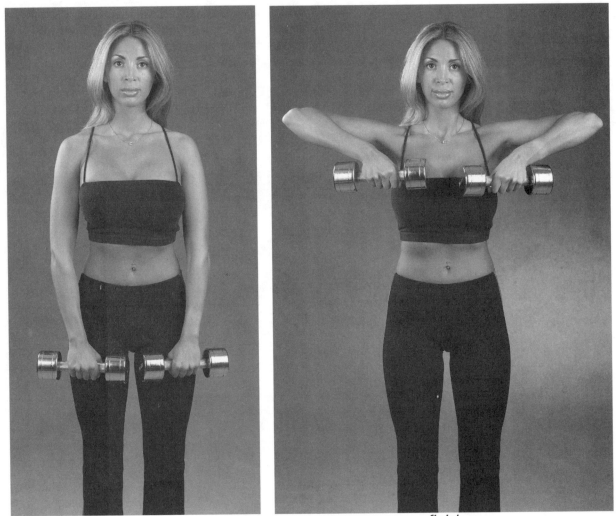

start   *finish*

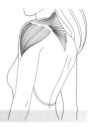

CABLE ROPE UPRIGHT ROW

Begin by taking a shoulder-width grip on a rope that is attached to a low cable pulley. Allow your arms to hang down from your shoulders and assume a comfortable stance with your knees slightly bent. Slowly pull the rope upward along the line of your body until your upper arm approaches shoulder level, keeping your elbows higher than your wrists at all times. Contract your delts and then slowly lower the rope along the same path back to the start position.

For Home Use:
Attach a strength band to a stationary object and perform the move as described. ▶

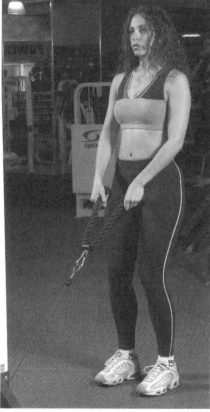

start

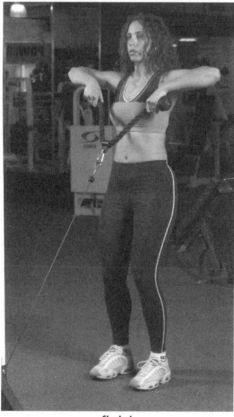

finish

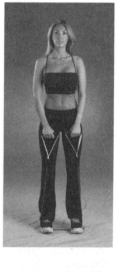

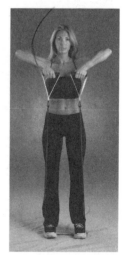

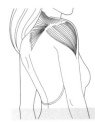

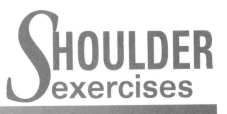

Group Three

Group Three exercises target the posterior (rear) head of the deltoid. This is accomplished by performing movements that employ horizontal extension of the shoulder joint (bringing your arm across and toward the back of your body). These maneuvers also work the infraspinatus and teres minor—two of the four "rotator cuff" muscles. Since the rotator cuff muscles are extremely important in stabilizing the shoulder joint, significant improvements in functional ability can be achieved.

Because it resides on the back of the body, the posterior deltoid is often overlooked. But just because you can't readily see this muscle doesn't mean that it isn't important. Functionally, the posterior delt provides stability to the shoulder joint. It counteracts the pull of the anterior deltoid, maintaining structural integrity of the joint. Moreover, from an aesthetic standpoint, it helps to balance out the other parts of the deltoid, improving the symmetry of your physique.

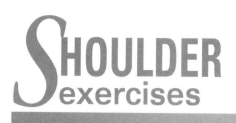
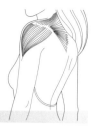

BENT LATERAL RAISE

Begin by grasping two dumbbells and bend your torso forward so that it is almost parallel with the ground. Allow the dumbbells to hang down in front of your body. With a slight bend to your elbows, raise the dumbbells up and out to the sides until your arms are parallel with the ground. Contract your delts at the top of the movement and then slowly return the dumbbells to the start position.

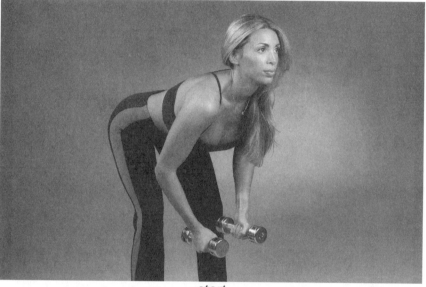

start

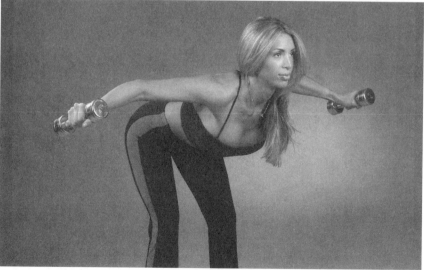

finish

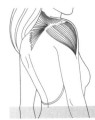

BENCH REAR LATERAL RAISE

Begin by grasping two dumbbells. Lie face down on an incline bench (adjusted to about a 30-degree incline) so that your torso is almost parallel with the ground. Allow the dumbbells to hang down in front of your body. With a slight bend to your elbows, raise the dumbbells up and out to the sides until your arms are parallel with the ground. Contract your delts at the top of the movement and then slowly return the dumbbells to the start position.

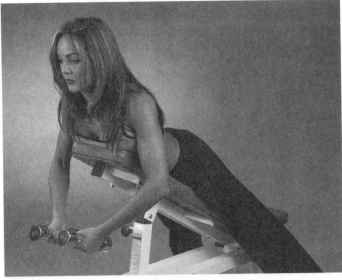

start

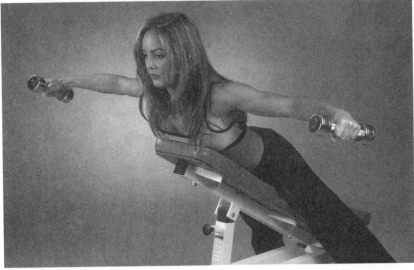

finish

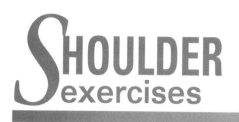

SHOULDER exercises

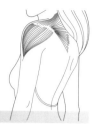

MACHINE REAR LATERAL RAISE

Begin by sitting face-forward in a pec deck apparatus. With a slight bend to your elbows, grasp the machine handles with your palms facing one another. Slowly pull the handles back in a semicircular arc as far as comfortably possible, keeping your arms parallel with the ground at all times. Contract your rear delts and then reverse direction, returning the handles to the start position.

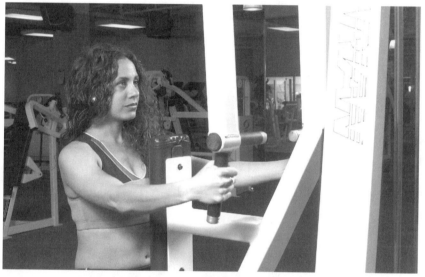

start

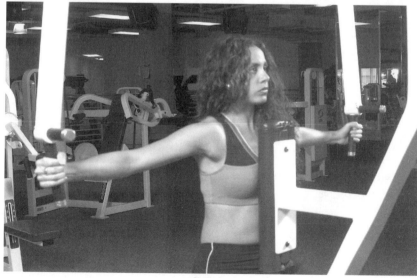

finish

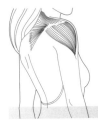

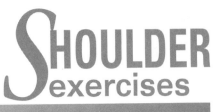

KNEELING CABLE BENT LATERAL RAISE

Begin by grasping a loop handle attached to a low pulley apparatus with your left hand and assume an "all-fours" position, stabilizing your torso with your right arm. With a slight bend to your elbow, raise the handle underneath your right arm, across your body, and up and out to the sides until it is parallel with the ground. Contract your delts at the top of the movement and then slowly return the handle to the start position. After completing the desired number of reps, repeat the process on your right side.

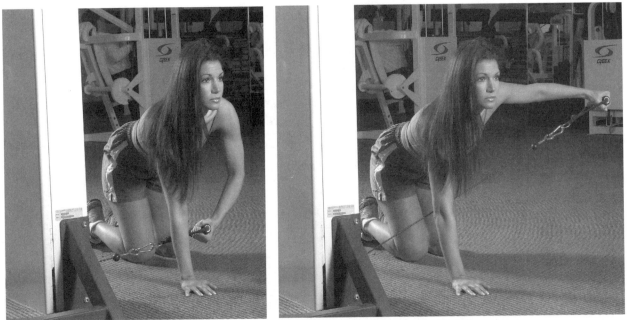

start   *finish*

For Home Use:
Attach a strength band to a stationary object and perform the move as described. ▶

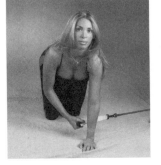 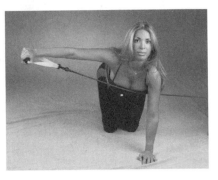

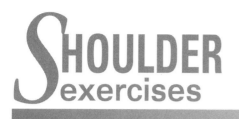
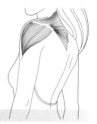

STANDING CABLE REAR LATERAL RAISE

Begin by grasping a loop handle attached to a high pulley apparatus with your left hand and stand so that your body faces forward. With a slight bend to your elbow, pull the handle across your body and out to your left side until you can't move it anymore. Contract your delts at the finish position and then slowly return the handle to the start position. After completing the desired number of reps, repeat the process on your right side.

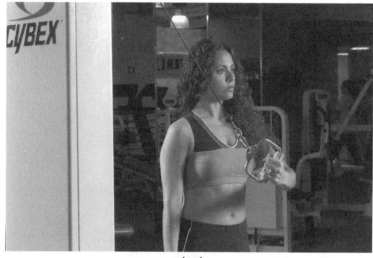

start

For Home Use:
Attach a strength band to a stationary object and perform the move as described. ▼

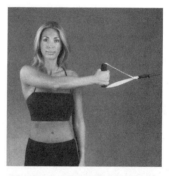

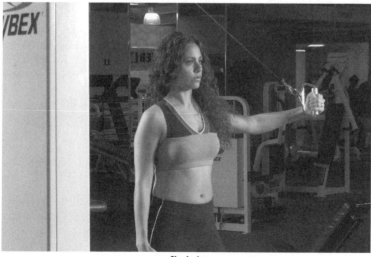

finish

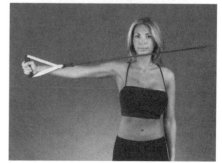

Table 5.1 summarizes the exercises for Sultry Shoulders.

TABLE 5.1

SUMMARY OF EXERCISES FOR SULTRY SHOULDERS

Group One	Group Two	Group Three
Dumbbell Shoulder Press	Dumbbell Lateral Raise	Bent Lateral Raise
Arnold Press	Cable Lateral Raise	Bench Rear Lateral Raise
Machine Shoulder Press	Machine Lateral Raise	Machine Rear Lateral Raise
Military Press	Dumbbell Upright Row	Kneeling Cable Bent Lateral Raise
Behind-the-Neck Press	Cable Rope Upright Row	Standing Cable Rear Lateral Raise

Sample Workouts

The following sample routines are provided for illustrative purposes. There are many other possibilities at your disposal, so be sure to experiment with different combinations.

Workout One

➠ Arnold Press
➠ Cable Rope Upright Row
➠ Machine Rear Lateral Raise

Workout Two

➠ Military Press
➠ Dumbbell Lateral Raise
➠ Kneeling Cable Bent Lateral Raise

Workout Three

➠ Machine Shoulder Press
➠ Cable Lateral Raise
➠ Bent Lateral Raise

Workout Four

➠ Machine Shoulder Press
➠ Dumbbell Upright Row
➠ Bench Rear Lateral Raise

SHAPELY CHEST

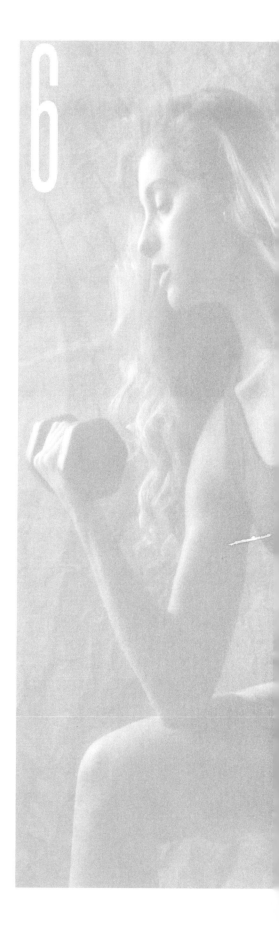

Is there any woman who doesn't want to firm up her chest? If so, I've yet to meet her!

Unfortunately, Mother Nature doesn't always cooperate with these wishes. Since breast tissue is predominantly comprised of fat, it succumbs to the forces of gravity and begins to sag over the years. Pregnancy and nursing only serve to make matters worse, causing the chest to droop even further. Unless something is done to counteract this phenomenon, it continues to "head south," sinking lower and lower as time goes by. Eventually, even a wonder-bra is of little help.

Since sleeveless attire is often low cut, the chest plays prominently in your ability to wear these outfits. It is a focal point of the body, giving contour and shape to your upper torso. And sleeveless often means braless, so your chest has to stand up on its own to meet the challenge.

Frequently, women seek a surgical solution to pump up their assets. Millions have gone under the knife, making breast augmentation one of the most popular of all cosmetic procedures. And without question, a little silicone or saline goes a long way to beefing up a bustline, providing almost immediate gratification for those willing to endure the process. In the hands of a good surgeon, results can be quite satisfactory.

But surgery does have its drawbacks. For one, the procedure is somewhat risky. Getting implants isn't like making a trip to the dentist. It is performed under general anesthesia, which in itself carries a certain degree of morbidity and mortality. In the post-surgical period, there is a good deal of pain and discomfort. The chest often remains swollen for weeks or even months, substantially limiting your functional ability.

There also are certain post-surgical dangers. Any time you put a foreign substance in your body, complications can arise. According to the Food and Drug Administration (FDA), up to 21 percent of healthy women require additional surgery to replace or remove their implants; 16 percent suffer breast pain; 10 percent lose sensation in their nipples; 9 percent develop hardening in the tissues around the nipples; and 5 percent experience leakage or deflation of the implant. Given these potential detriments, implants definitely aren't for everyone. Needless to say, before a decision of this magnitude is made, you must weigh all the pros and cons.

The good news is, exercise can provide a natural alternative to cosmetic surgery. When properly implemented, a well-designed training routine can help to offset the ravages of time and restore your chest to its previous glory. Although it won't directly increase your cup size (breast tissue is fat and, as previously discussed, fat cannot be shaped), targeted bodysculpting lifts and defines your chest, giving it a fuller, shapelier appearance (yes, you actually can defy gravity!). So for those who don't want to go through the rigors of surgery or prefer to remain "au naturel" for philosophical reasons, take heart; if you're willing to put in the effort, results are guaranteed.

How is this possible? Well, the breasts are supported by a vast network of muscles and connective tissue—structures that respond to targeted exercise. By utilizing different movements and training at a variety of angles, you can target various parts of the chest to achieve complete development. For example, rounding out the upper pectoral region gives fullness to the bustline; adding to the middle aspect enhances the overall shape of the chest; and developing the inner portion creates the illusion of cleavage. With an understanding of basic bodysculpting techniques, a multitude of possibilities are at your disposal.

Anatomy of the Chest

The chest is comprised of the pectorals (pecs, for short). Let's take a look at the form and function of each muscle:

⟶ The ***pectoralis major*** is a large, sunburst-shaped muscle that has two heads. The clavicular head originates on the front of the clavicle (collarbone) while the sternocostal head originates on the manubrium (top of the sternum) as well as the upper six ribs. Both heads attach to the humerus (upper arm bone) and have similar functions in shoulder joint adduction (bringing the arm toward the midline of the body) and medial rotation of the upper arm. Because of their different origins, however, each head also has its own unique function. Namely, the clavicular head helps to flex the shoulder joint while the sternocostal head helps to extend it.

➠ The ***pectoralis minor*** is a small, strap-like muscle. It originates on the third, fourth and fifth ribs and inserts on the coracoid process of the scapula (shoulder blade). While its main function is scapular depression, it also assists the pectoralis major by abducting the scapula during various chest movements.

Figure 6.1 provides an anatomical diagram that shows the location of the pectoral muscles.

FIGURE 6.1
Pectoral Muscles

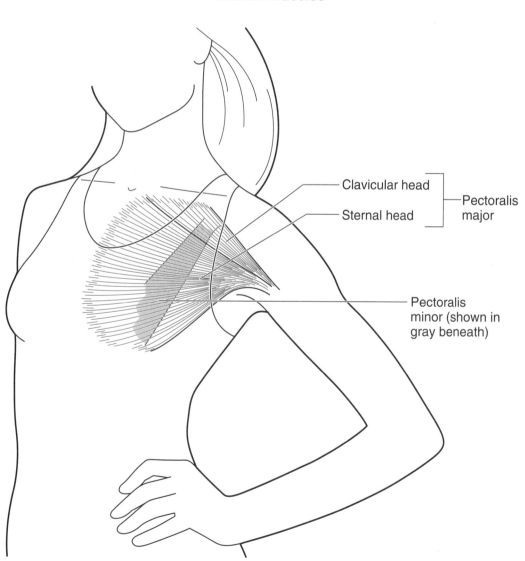

Clavicular head ⎫
Sternal head ⎬ Pectoralis major

Pectoralis minor (shown in gray beneath)

Chest "Dos and Don'ts"

The following points should be kept in mind during chest training.

➠ ***Don't*** *put your feet up on the bench during chest training.* Many women feel more comfortable keeping their feet on the bench when performing chest exercises. This, however, reduces the natural lumbar curvature of the spine, increasing pressure on the lower back. Additionally, stability while lifting is impaired, increasing your risk of losing balance, especially when struggling to complete the last few reps of a set.

➠ ***Do*** *keep your feet planted firmly on the floor.* Make sure they remain grounded throughout the entire set.

➠ ***Don't*** *allow your butt to rise up during chest training.* In order to complete a difficult repetition, a woman will often lift her butt off the bench. But while this may help to improve leverage, it also reduces the amount of stress applied to the pectoral muscles. What's more, the lower back is placed in a precarious position, heightening the potential for injury.

➠ ***Do*** *keep your butt pressed to the bench.* Use only the target muscles to lift the weight and avoid any extraneous movement of the lower body or torso.

➠ ***Don't*** *let your elbows come close to your body during chest training.* Most women give little regard to the position of their arms during the performance of chest exercises. But when your elbows approach your sides, the chest muscles slacken. Hence, they lose some of their force-generating capacity, leading to decreased results.

➠ ***Do*** *keep your elbows flared out to the sides at all times.* They should form a right angle with your body at the start of each rep.

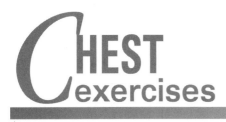

CHEST exercises

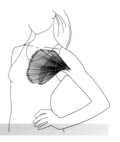

Group One

Group One exercises target the upper (clavicular) pectoral region. This is accomplished by performing compound movements where the upper pecs directly oppose gravity. Developing this portion of the chest gives a lift to the breasts, helping to counteract the effects of gravity.

Patience and persistence are necessary to achieve the desired development of the upper chest. Since there isn't much muscle in the area (as compared to the middle portion), it responds rather slowly to exercise. Complicating matters, the anterior deltoids become increasingly active during the performance of these movements, reducing the amount of stimulation to the clavicular head.

For optimal results, it's beneficial to prioritize these exercises and perform them first in your chest routine. Your strength levels will then be at their peak, allowing you to give each rep your all. Further, make sure that the bench incline doesn't exceed 30 degrees. This will minimize shoulder involvement and thereby keep most of the stress on the upper chest.

Group 1

INCLINE DUMBBELL PRESS (page 58)

INCLINE MACHINE CHEST PRESS (page 59)

BENCH PUSH-UP (page 60)

EXER-BALL DUMBBELL PRESS (page 61)

INCLINE BARBELL PRESS (page 62)

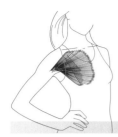 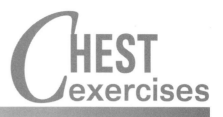

INCLINE DUMBBELL PRESS

Begin by lying face up on an incline bench, planting your feet firmly on the floor. Grasp two dumbbells and, with your palms facing away from your body, bring them to shoulder level so that they rest just above your armpits. Simultaneously press both dumbbells directly over your chest, moving them in toward each other on the ascent. At the finish of the movement, the sides of the dumbbells should gently touch together. Feel a contraction in your chest muscles and then slowly reverse direction, returning to the start position.

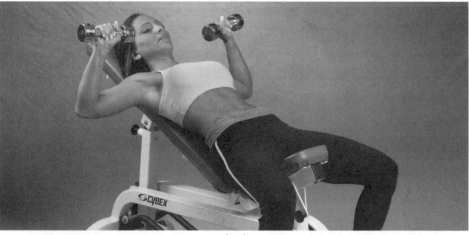

start

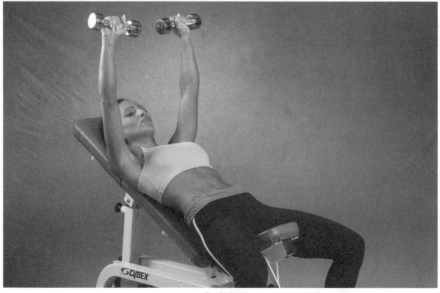

finish

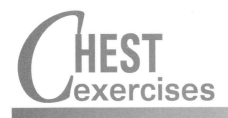

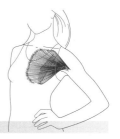

INCLINE MACHINE CHEST PRESS

Begin by sitting in an incline chest press machine, aligning your upper chest with the handles on the machine. Grasp the handles with a shoulder-width grip, keeping your palms facing away from your body. Slowly press the handles forward, stopping just before you fully lock out your elbows. Feel a contraction in your chest muscles at the finish of the movement and then slowly reverse direction, returning to the start position.

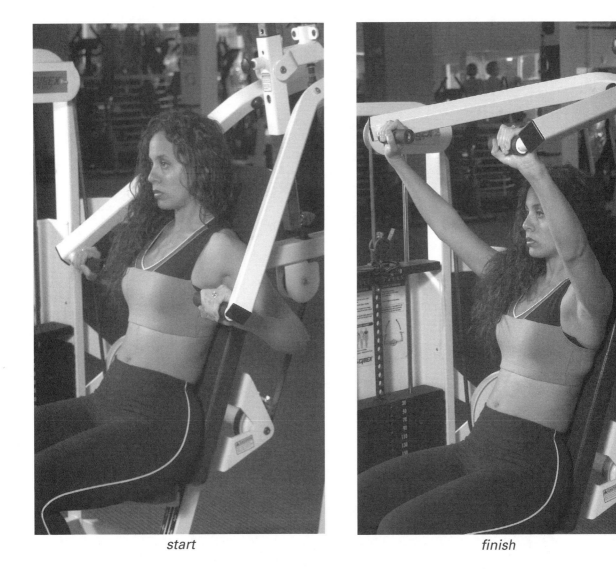

start   *finish*

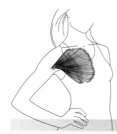
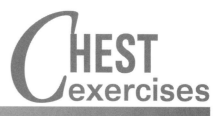
BENCH PUSH-UP

Begin with your hands on the floor and feet up on a flat bench. Your torso and legs should remain rigid, keeping your back perfectly straight throughout the move. Bend your arms and slowly lower your body downward, stopping just before your upper chest touches the ground. Feel a stretch in your chest muscles and then reverse direction, pushing your body up along the same path back to the start position.

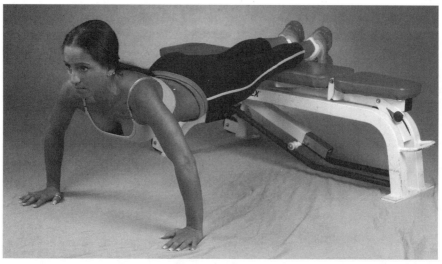

start

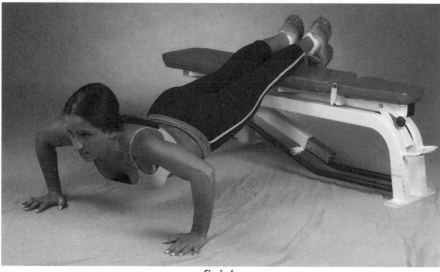

finish

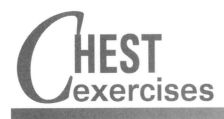

CHEST exercises

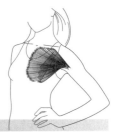

EXER-BALL DUMBBELL PRESS

Lie back on an exercise ball with your feet planted firmly on the floor. Grasp two dumbbells and, with your palms facing away from your body, bring them to shoulder level so that they rest just above your armpits. Simultaneously press both dumbbells directly over your chest, moving them in toward each other on the ascent. At the finish of the movement, the sides of the dumbbells should gently touch together. Feel a contraction in your chest muscles at the top of the movement and then slowly reverse direction, returning to the start position.

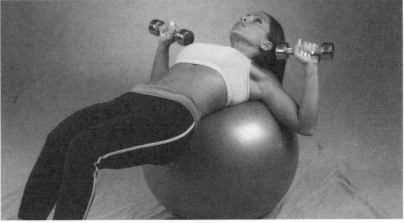

start

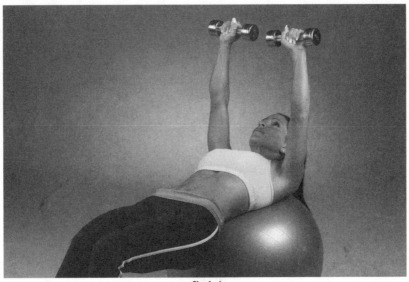

finish

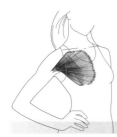
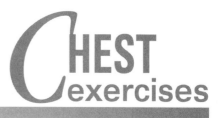
INCLINE BARBELL PRESS

Begin by lying face up on an incline bench set at approximately 30 to 40 degrees, planting your feet firmly on the floor. Grasp a barbell with a shoulder-width grip and bring it down to the upper aspect of your chest. Press the bar directly over your chest, moving it in a straight line into the air. Feel a contraction in your chest muscles at the top of the movement and then slowly reverse direction, returning to the start position.

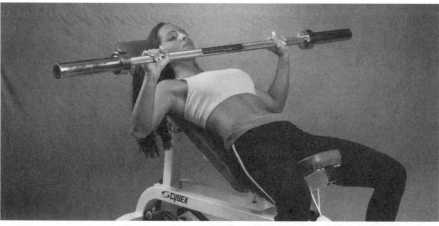

start

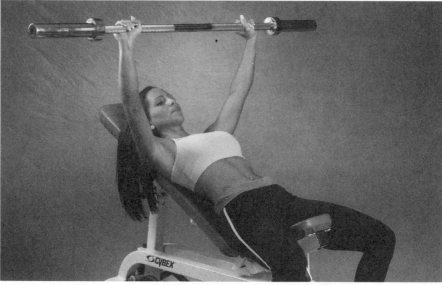

finish

CHEST exercises

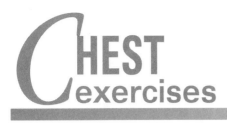
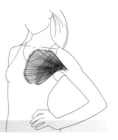

Group Two

Group Two exercises focus on the lower and middle (sternocostal) pectoral regions. This is accomplished by using compound movements where the sternocostal portion of the chest is put in a position to directly oppose gravity. Attention to this area helps to augment the shape of breasts, creating the illusion of a bigger bust.

The middle chest is rather "meaty" and therefore develops quite readily. Most women will see results in a relatively short period of time. You therefore must be careful that development of this region doesn't overshadow that of the upper chest. If an imbalance exists, perform these movements last in the giant set in order to mitigate further development.

During exercise performance, make sure to avoid locking out your elbows when you reach the finish position. When your joints are fully extended, stress to the target muscles is diminished and the potential for joint-related injury is increased. Consequently, stop just short of a full lockout, keeping constant tension on the pecs at all times.

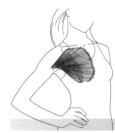

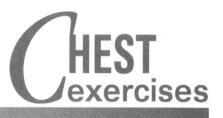

FLAT DUMBBELL PRESS

Begin by lying face-up on a flat bench with your feet planted firmly on the floor. Grasp two dumbbells and, with your palms facing away from your body, bring them to shoulder level so that they rest just above your armpits. Simultaneously press both dumbbells directly over your chest, moving them in toward each other on the ascent. At the finish of the movement, the sides of the dumbbells should gently touch together. Feel a contraction in your chest muscles at the top of the movement and then slowly reverse direction, returning to the start position.

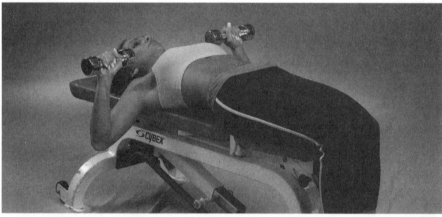

start

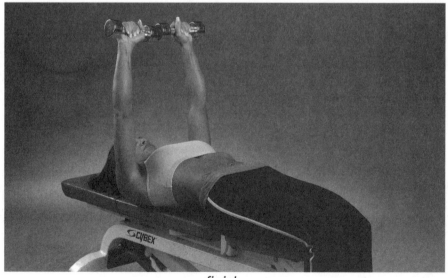

finish

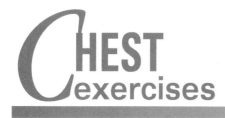

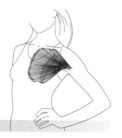

MACHINE CHEST PRESS

Begin by sitting in a chest press machine, aligning your upper chest with the handles on the machine. Grasp the handles with a shoulder-width grip, keeping your palms facing away from your body. Slowly press the handles forward, stopping just before you fully lock out your elbows. Feel a contraction in your chest muscles at the finish of the movement and then slowly reverse direction, returning to the start position.

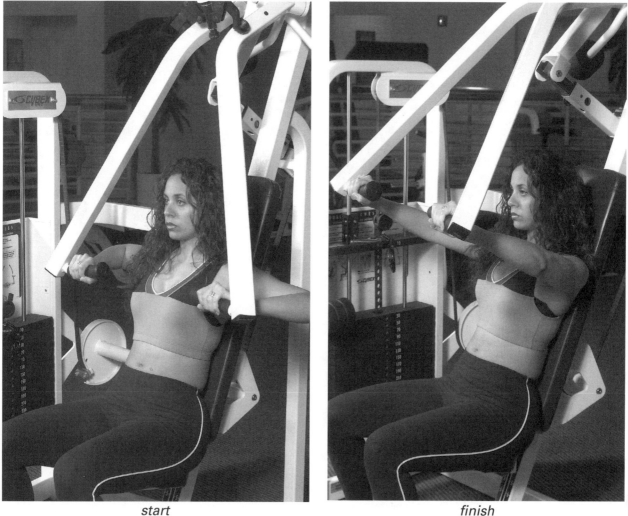

start   *finish*

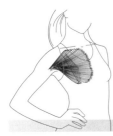
FLAT BARBELL PRESS

Begin by lying face-up on a flat bench with your feet planted firmly on the floor. Grasp a barbell and, with your palms facing away from your body, lower the bar so that it rests just above your breasts. Press the bar upward in a straight line over your chest, stopping just short of locking out your elbows. Feel a contraction in your chest muscles at the top of the movement and then slowly reverse direction, returning to the start position.

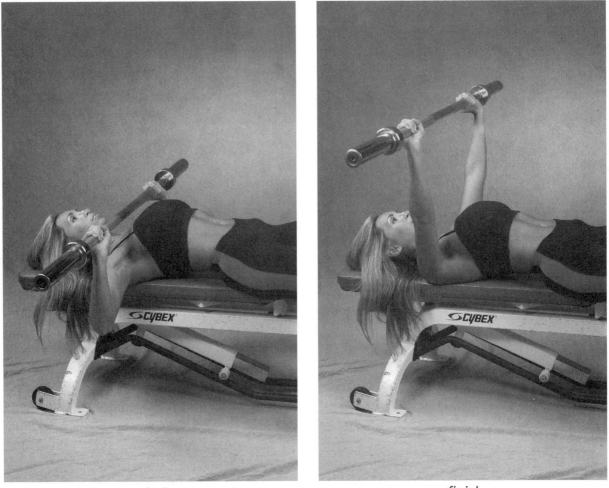

start   *finish*

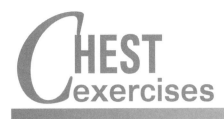

CHEST exercises

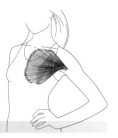

PUSH-UP

Begin with your hands and knees on the floor. Your torso and legs should remain rigid, keeping your back perfectly straight throughout the move. Bend your arms and slowly lower your body downward, stopping just before your chest touches the ground. Feel a stretch in your chest muscles and then reverse direction, pushing your body up along the same path back to the start position.

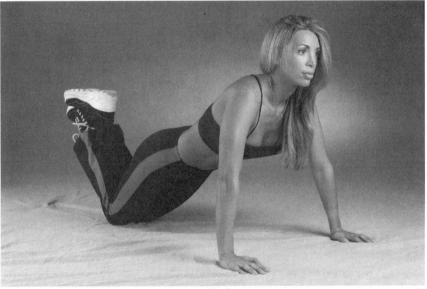

start

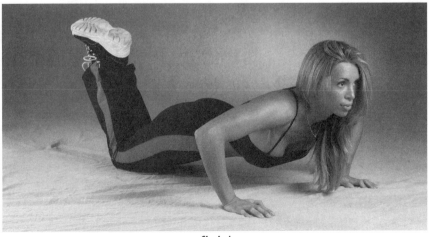

finish

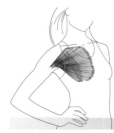

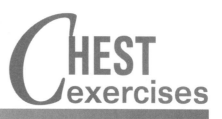

CHEST DIP

Begin by grasping the bars on a parallel bar apparatus with your palms facing in toward each other. Bend your legs at a 90-degree angle, cross your ankles, and tilt your upper body forward with your hips to the rear. Maintaining a distinct forward tilt, slowly bend your elbows and lower your body as far as comfortably possible. Then, slowly reverse direction and return to the start position. If you need assistance, you can have a partner hold your ankles and spot you during performance. Alternatively, you can use a Gravitron® machine, which provides mechanical assistance in the execution of the move.

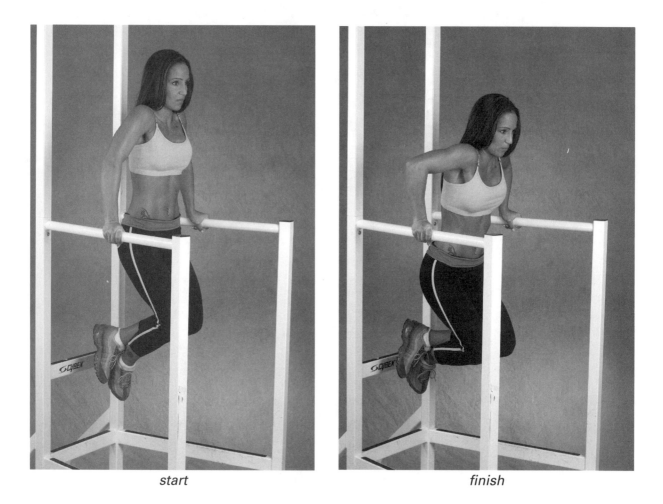

start   *finish*

CHEST exercises

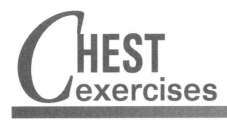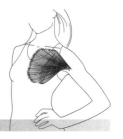

Group Three

Group Three exercises help to isolate the pectoral muscles. This is accomplished by performing single-joint movements where your arms are brought across the midline of your body (a maneuver called *horizontal adduction*). Although other muscles are involved during performance, their contribution is significantly less than in compound movements. Consequently, better pectoral isolation can be attained and the potential for bodysculpting is thereby enhanced.

Technique is extremely important in these moves. One of the biggest mistakes that people make is to straighten the elbows during performance. Doing so, however, only serves to turn the exercise into a pressing movement. The triceps in turn become increasingly active, taking stress away from the target muscles of the chest.

For best results, maintain a slight bend at the elbow and keep the arms rigid throughout each rep. Lift the weights in a rounded motion (as if you're hugging a tree or a beach ball), making sure that the pecs do the majority of the work.

It's also important to avoid stretching back too far at the beginning of these moves. If a joint is stretched beyond its capacity, you run the risk of damaging connective tissue. To avoid this fate, stay within a comfortable range, stretching only to where your flexibility will allow. With rare exception, your upper arm should never go below the plane of your upper torso; any further, and the chance for injury is significantly increased.

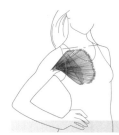
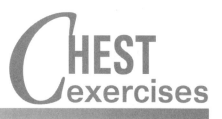
INCLINE DUMBBELL FLYE

Begin by lying back on an incline bench set at approximately 30 to 40 degrees, planting your feet firmly on the floor. Grasp two dumbbells and bring them out to your sides, maintaining a slight bend to your elbows throughout the move. Your palms should be facing in and toward the ceiling, and your upper arms should be roughly parallel with the level of the bench. Slowly raise the weights upward in a circular motion, as if you were hugging a large tree. Gently touch the weights together at the top of the move and, after feeling a contraction in your chest muscles, slowly return the weights along the same path to the start position.

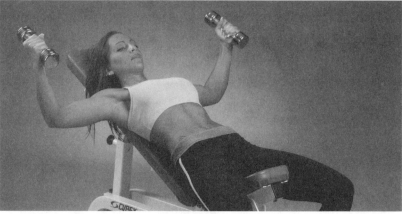

start

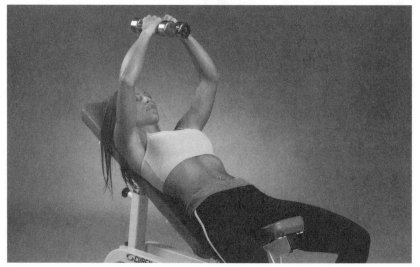

finish

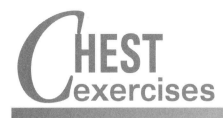

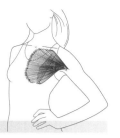

CHEST exercises

FLAT DUMBBELL FLYE

Begin by lying back on a flat bench, planting your feet firmly on the floor. Grasp two dumbbells and bring them out to your sides, maintaining a slight bend to your elbows throughout the move. Your palms should be facing in and toward the ceiling, and your upper arms should be roughly parallel with the level of the bench. Slowly raise the weights upward in a semicircular motion, as if you were hugging a large tree. Gently touch the weights together at the top of the move and, after feeling a contraction in your chest muscles, slowly return the weights along the same path to the start position.

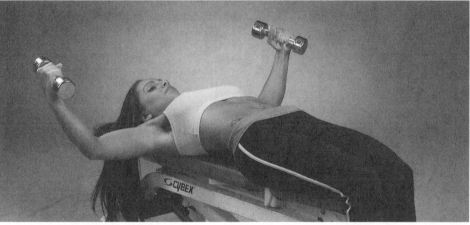

start

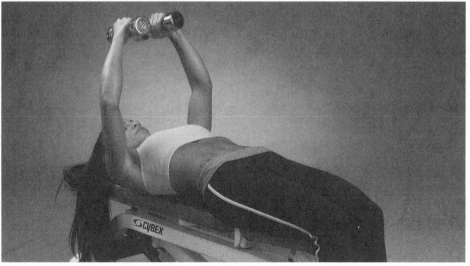

finish

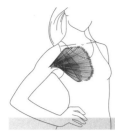 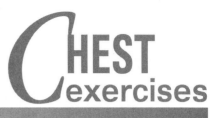

PEC DECK

Begin by placing your forearms on the pads of a pec deck machine. Your elbows should be pressed into the pads at all times and your back should remain immobile throughout the movement. Simultaneously press both pads together, allowing them to gently touch each other directly in front of your chest. Hold this position for a count of two while contracting your chest muscles and then slowly reverse direction, returning to the start position.

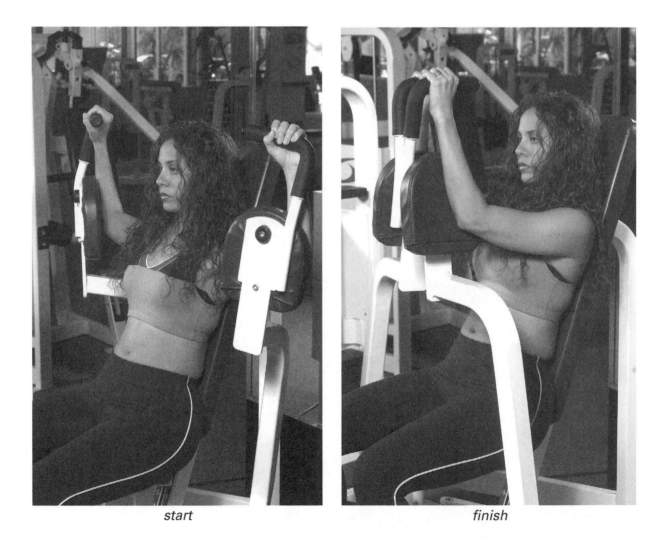

start   finish

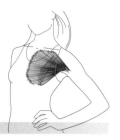

CHEST exercises

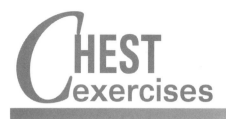

HIGH PULLEY CABLE CROSSOVER

Begin by grasping the handles of an overhead pulley apparatus (cable crossover machine). Stand with your feet about shoulder-width apart and your torso bent slightly forward at the waist. Slowly pull both handles downward and across your body, creating a semicircular movement. Bring your hands together at the level of your hips and squeeze your chest muscles so that you feel a contraction in the cleavage area. Then slowly reverse direction, allowing your hands to return along the same path to the start position.

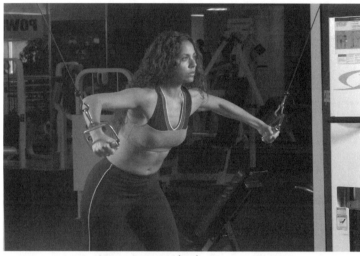

start

For Home Use:
Attach a strength band to a stationary object and perform the move as described. ▼

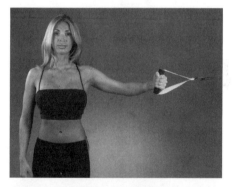

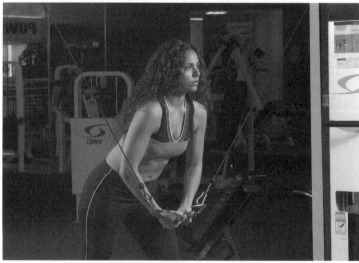

finish

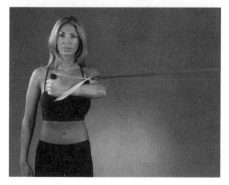

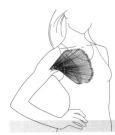

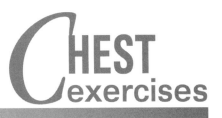

Low Pulley Cable Crossover

Begin by grasping the loop handles of a low pulley apparatus (cable crossover machine). Stand with your feet about shoulder-width apart and your torso bent slightly forward at the waist. Slowly pull both handles up and across your body, creating a semi-circular movement. Bring your hands together at the level of your hips and squeeze your chest muscles so that you feel a contraction in the cleavage area. Then slowly reverse direction, allowing your hands to return along the same path to the start position.

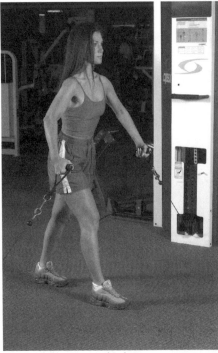
start

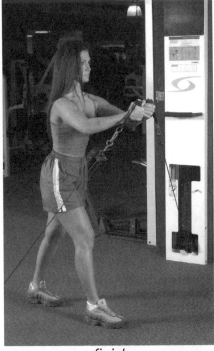
finish

For Home Use:
Attach a strength band to a stationary object and perform the move as described. ▶

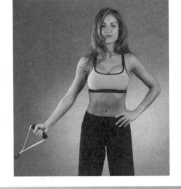

Table 6.1 summarizes the exercises for a Shapely Chest.

TABLE 6.1
SUMMARY OF EXERCISES FOR A SHAPELY CHEST

Group One	Group Two	Group Three
Incline Dumbbell Press	Flat Dumbbell Press	Incline Dumbbell Flye
Incline Machine Chest Press	Machine Chest Press	Flat Dumbbell Flye
Bench Push-up	Flat Barbell Press	Pec Deck
Exer-ball Dumbbell Press	Push-up	High Pulley Cable Crossover
Incline Barbell Press	Chest Dip	Low Pulley Cable Crossover

Sample Workouts

The following sample routines are provided for illustrative purposes. There are many other possibilities at your disposal, so be sure to experiment with different combinations.

Workout One

➡ Incline Dumbbell Press
➡ Push-up
➡ Flat Dumbbell Flye

Workout Two

➡ Incline Machine Chest Press
➡ Flat Dumbbell Press
➡ Low Pulley Cable Crossover

Workout Three

➡ Bench Push-up
➡ Chest Dip
➡ Pec Deck

Workout Four

➡ Incline Machine Chest Press
➡ Machine Chest Press
➡ Incline Dumbbell Flye

TERRIFIC TRICEPS

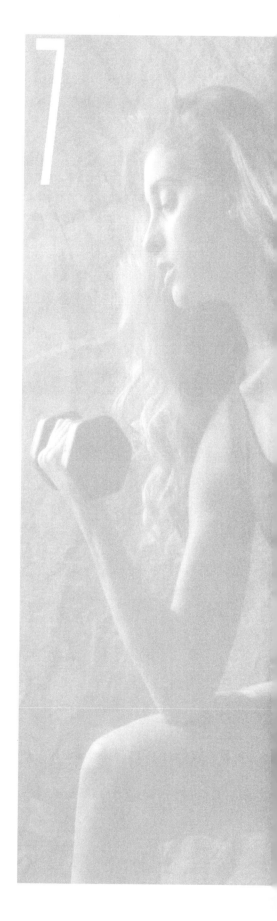

Of all the upper body regions, it's the triceps that tend to give women the most grief. Like the hips and thighs in the lower body, this area often is a real trouble spot. The quandary here is twofold: too much body fat and too little muscle.

The accumulation of fat around the triceps is largely physiologic in origin. For untold reasons, women just have a predisposition to store fat in this region. It's as if the triceps are a magnet to fat, attracting any extra adipose that doesn't settle in the lower body.

From a muscular perspective, the triceps present additional problems. Occupying about 60 percent of the lean upper arm mass, it's only slightly larger in diameter than the biceps. Thus, its relatively small stature doesn't provide a great deal of support to the region.

This double-whammy only gets worse with age. With an abundance of fat and declining amounts of muscle, you end up with loose, flabby triceps that have no shape or definition. And because the area directly opposes gravity, there is nothing to stop it from sagging. Ultimately, your poor arms just hang down like bat wings when held out to the sides; not a pretty sight, by any stretch of the imagination.

Adding insult to injury, cellulite can sometimes invade the backs of the arms. Cellulite is a genetic condition—you either have it or you don't. It is due to the composition of human skin, which has three fundamental layers. The top layer is comprised of a cellular-based tissue called the *dermis*. Its primary purpose is to protect your body from outside contaminants. The lower layer is made up of adipose tissue—plain old fat. It has several functions including insulating the body, padding the internal organs and providing a source of long-term energy. Between these two layers is a fibrous sheet of connective tissue called *superficial fascia*. It is substantially thicker than the dermis and acts like an internal stocking to support the skin and hold down the underlying adipose tissue.

How does this relate to cellulite? Well, in some women, the superficial fascia in the triceps region is irregular and discontinuous, forming honeycomb-like patterns beneath the dermis. Hence, when fat accumulates, it pushes up toward the skin's surface in clusters, giving the skin a lumpy, dimpled appearance.

If getting your arms into shape is beginning to seem hopeless, take heart. Your triceps can, and will, respond to dedicated exercise. Despite its small size, the triceps tend to firm up quite nicely. As muscle tone increases, your arms begin to take shape and display a symmetrical appearance.

Now it's important to realize that targeted triceps training won't directly whittle away stored arm fat (remember, you can't spot reduce!). But as you continue to work out and eat right, unwanted adipose will gradually disappear. Better yet, any cellulite will also diminish. Lean muscle tone helps to smooth underlying fat, making dimples less evident. Once body fat is reduced to acceptable levels, your triceps will be taut and toned and you'll be able to hold out your arms with complete confidence in any sleeveless outfit!

Anatomy of the Triceps

The bottom portion of the upper arm is comprised of the triceps. Let's take a look at the form and function of this muscle.

The ***triceps brachii*** is comprised of three distinct heads, each joining to form a common tendon that attaches to the ulna (one of the bones in the forearm) but having separate points of origin. The lateral head originates on the outer portion of the humerus (upper arm bone) and the medial head originates on the middle portion of the humerus (it lies deep and between the other two heads and thus is mostly hidden from direct view); neither of these heads crosses the shoulder joint. The long head originates at the scapula (shoulder blade), just inferior to the head of the humerus at the shoulder joint. All three heads of the triceps function to extend the elbow. Because the long head crosses the glenohumeral joint, it also is involved in various movements relating to the shoulder.

Figure 7.1 provides an anatomical diagram that shows the location of the triceps muscles.

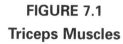

FIGURE 7.1
Triceps Muscles

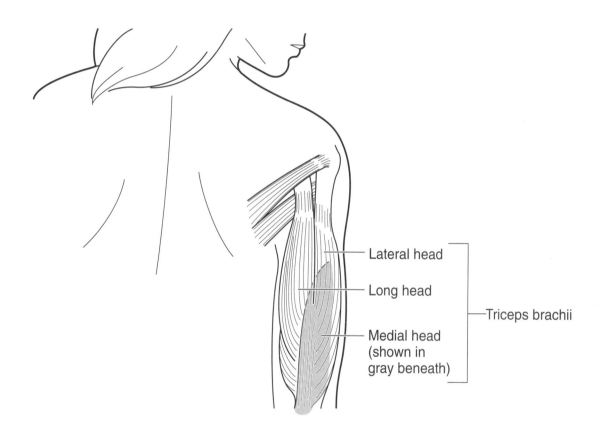

Triceps "Dos and Don'ts"

The following points should be kept in mind during triceps training.

➡ ***Don't*** *flare your elbows during triceps training.* There is a natural tendency to bring the elbows away from the body when working the triceps. Flaring the elbows allows the chest to become increasingly active, providing increased force capacity and thereby making the move easier to complete. But the downside is that the triceps assumes a secondary role in performance. Since the chest is infinitely more powerful than the much smaller triceps, the ultimate effect is to reduce triceps development.

➡ ***Do*** *keep your elbows close to your body at all times.* This will keep the focus on the triceps and reduce involvement from other muscle groups.

➡ ***Don't*** *allow your upper arms to move during triceps training.* In order to complete a rep, it is common to bring the upper arm downward. This, however, brings the scapular muscles into play, taking stress away from the triceps.

➡ ***Do*** *keep your upper arms perfectly still throughout each exercise.* The forearm is the only thing that should move during performance, without assistance from ancillary muscles.

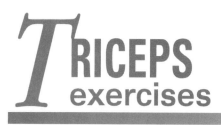

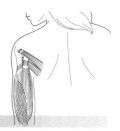

TRICEPS exercises

Group One

Group One exercises target the long head of the triceps—the muscle that lies at the bottom-most portion of the upper arm. This is accomplished by keeping your shoulder flexed throughout each move (i.e., your arm is raised and your elbow points toward the ceiling). Since the long head crosses the shoulder joint, it becomes stretched in shoulder flexion and therefore can exert more force than the other two heads.

The long head of the triceps is extremely important from an aesthetic standpoint. If it lacks tone, you end up with drooping arms that seemingly flap in the wind when held out to the sides (the bat-wing syndrome). This effect is apparent even in the absence of a significant amount of body fat in the region. Only by developing the long head will you offset the loose skin look and make the area firm and hard.

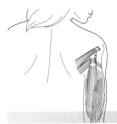

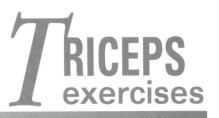

ONE-ARM OVERHEAD DUMBBELL EXTENSION

Begin by grasping a dumbbell in your right hand with your feet firmly planted on the floor. Bend your elbow and allow the weight to hang down behind your head as far as comfortably possible. Slowly straighten your arm, keeping your elbow back and pointed toward the ceiling throughout the move. Contract your triceps and then slowly lower the weight along the same path back to the start position. After you have performed the desired number of reps, repeat the process on your left.

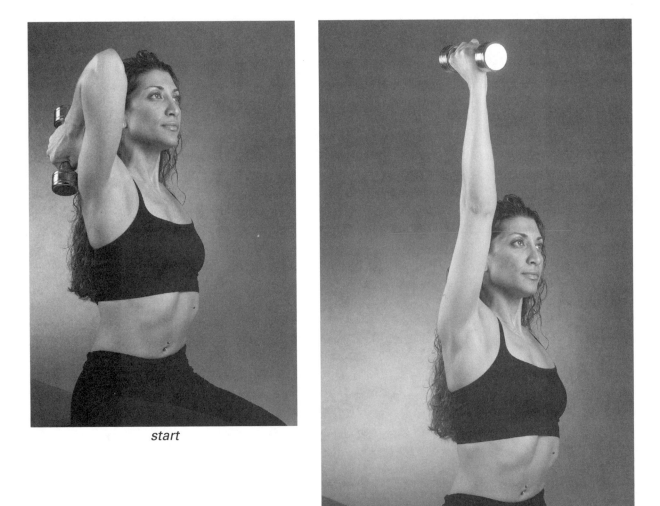

start

finish

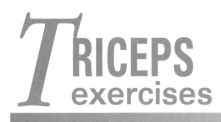 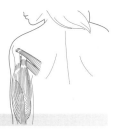

TRICEPS exercises

TWO-ARM OVERHEAD DUMBBELL EXTENSION

Begin by grasping the stem of a dumbbell with both hands. Bend your elbows and allow the weight to hang down behind your head as far as comfortably possible. Slowly straighten your arms, keeping your elbows back and pointed toward the ceiling throughout the move. Contract your triceps and then slowly lower the weight along the same path back to the start position.

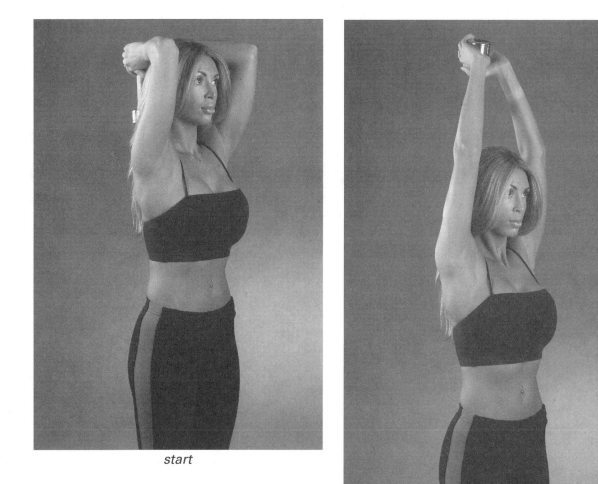

start

finish

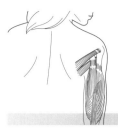

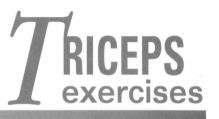

SEATED OVERHEAD CABLE EXTENSION

Begin by sitting on a bench with your back to a cable pulley apparatus. Grasp a bar attached to the pulley apparatus with your palms facing away from your body. Keeping your elbows at your ears, bend your elbows and allow your hands to hang down behind your head as far as comfortably possible. Slowly straighten your arms, keeping your elbows back throughout the move. Contract your triceps and then slowly lower the weight along the same path back to the start position.

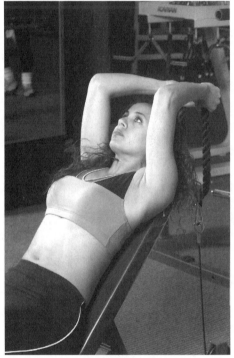

start

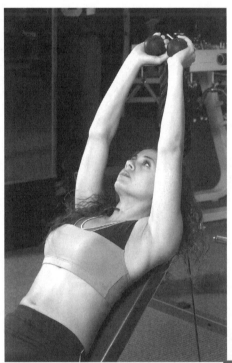

finish

For Home Use:

Attach a strength band to a stationary object and perform the move as described. ▶

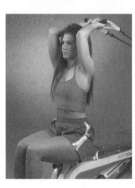

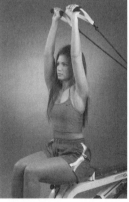

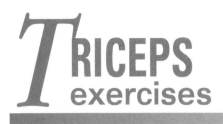

TRICEPS exercises

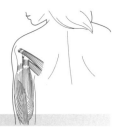

STANDING OVERHEAD ROPE EXTENSION

Begin by turning your body away from a low cable pulley apparatus. Bend your torso forward and grasp a rope attached to the pulley apparatus with your palms facing each other. Keeping your elbows at your ears, bend your elbows and allow your hands to hang down behind your head as far as comfortably possible. Slowly straighten your arms, keeping your elbows back throughout the move. Contract your triceps and then slowly lower the weight along the same path back to the start position.

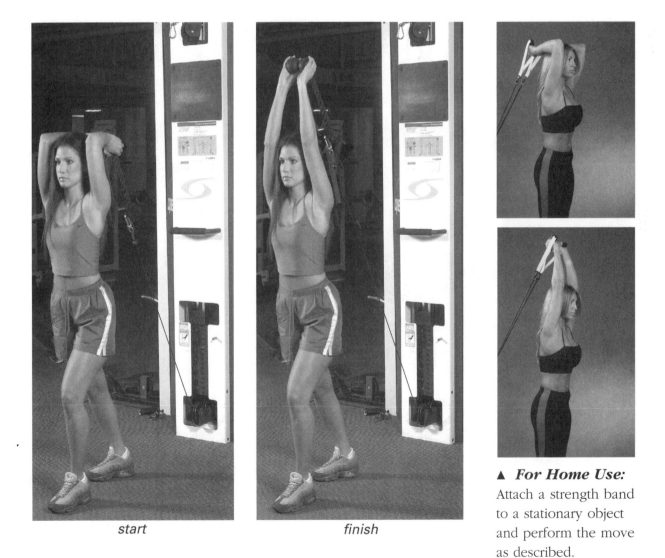

start　　　　　　　　*finish*

▲ *For Home Use:* Attach a strength band to a stationary object and perform the move as described.

SEATED OVERHEAD EZ-CURL EXTENSION

Begin by grasping an EZ-curl bar with your palms facing away from your body. Bend your elbows and allow the bar to hang down behind your head as far as comfortably possible. Slowly straighten your arms, keeping your elbows back and pointed toward the ceiling throughout the move. Contract your triceps and then slowly lower the bar along the same path back to the start position.

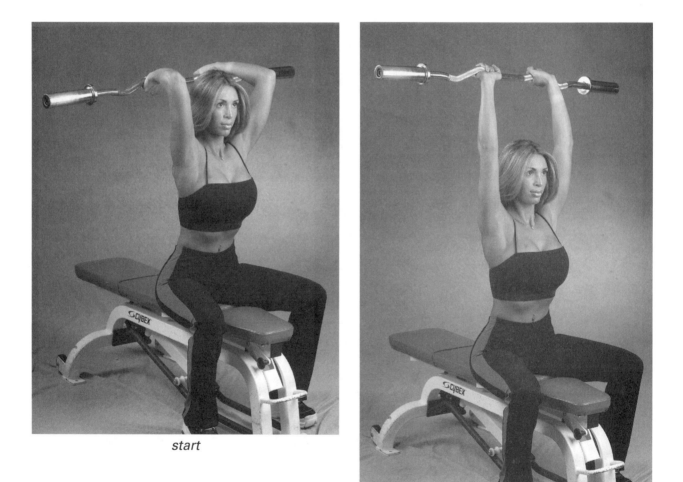

start

finish

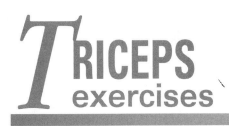RICEPS exercises

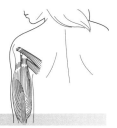

Group Two

Group Two exercises emphasize the medial and lateral heads of the triceps. This is accomplished by performing movements with the upper arms extended at your sides. Doing so renders the long head less active, which in turn allows the other two heads to accomplish a greater amount of work. When the upper arms are slightly hyperextended (brought behind the torso), the effect is even more pronounced and even better isolation is achieved.

Both the lateral and medial heads combine to delineate the middle region of the upper arm, helping to form the distinctive "horseshoe" appearance of the triceps. The lateral head, in particular, creates the "tail" of the horseshoe. When properly developed, this gives the triceps a polished look that is a sure sign your arms are in peak condition.

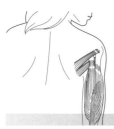
ROPE PRESSDOWN

Begin by grasping a rope that is attached to a high pulley apparatus with an overhand grip. Assume a shoulder-width stance with your knees slightly bent and your torso angled forward. Bend your arms so that your elbows form a 90-degree angle. Keeping your elbows in at your sides, slowly straighten your arms. Contract your triceps and then reverse direction and return to the start position.

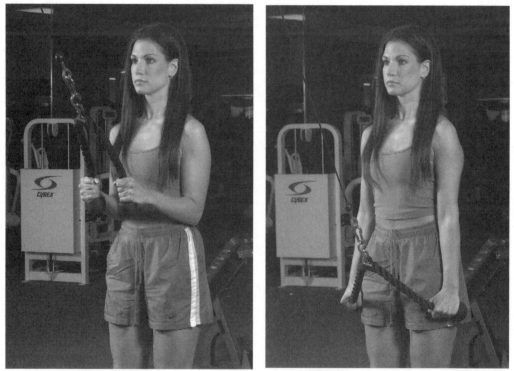

start   *finish*

For Home Use:
Attach a strength band to a stationary object and perform the move as described. ▶

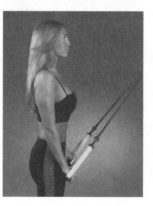
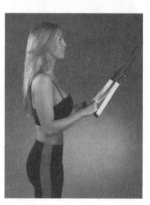

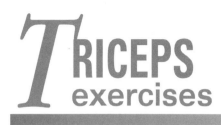

TRICEPS exercises

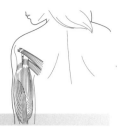

DUMBBELL KICKBACK

Begin by standing with your torso bent forward so that it is virtually parallel with the ground. Grasp a dumbbell with your right hand and press your right arm against your side with your elbow bent at 90-degree angles. With your palm facing your body, raise the weight by straightening your arm until it is parallel with the floor. Then, reverse direction and return the weight to the start position. After finishing the desired number of repetitions, repeat the process on your left.

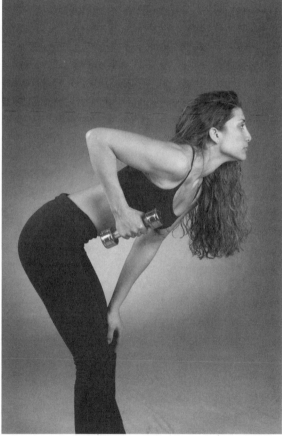

start

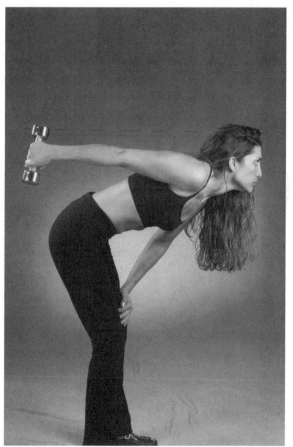

finish

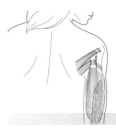 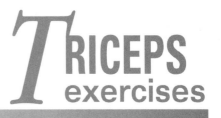

TRICEPS BENCH DIP

Begin by placing your heels on the floor and your hands on the edge of a flat bench, keeping your arms straight. Slowly bend your elbows as far as comfortably possible, allowing your butt to descend below the level of the bench. Make sure your elbows stay close to your body throughout the move. Then, reverse direction and straighten your arms, returning to the start position.

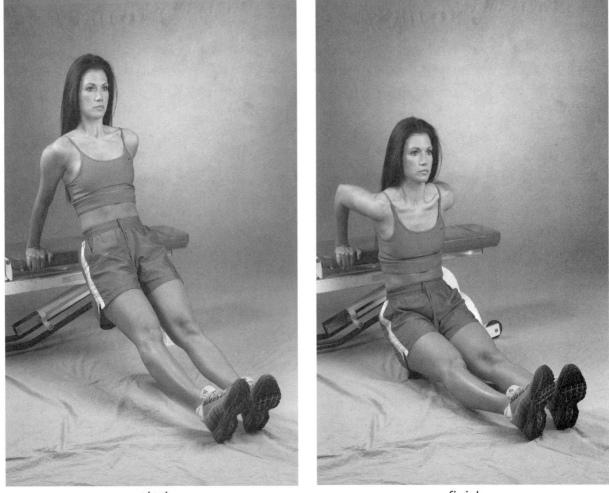

start   finish

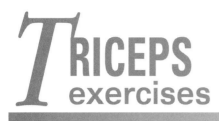

TRICEPS exercises

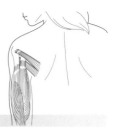

ONE-ARM REVERSE PRESSDOWN

Begin by grasping a loop handle that is attached to a high pulley apparatus with your left hand, palm facing up. Assume a shoulder-width stance with your knees slightly bent and your torso angled forward. Bend your arm so that your elbow forms a 90-degree angle. Keeping your elbow in at your side, slowly straighten your left arm. Contract your triceps and then reverse direction and return to the start position. After performing the desired number of repetitions, repeat the process on your right.

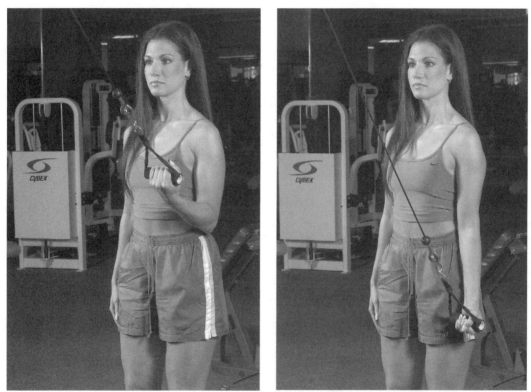

start   *finish*

For Home Use:
Attach a strength band to a stationary object and perform the move as described. ▶

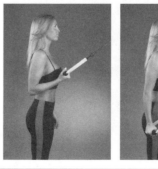

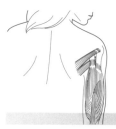 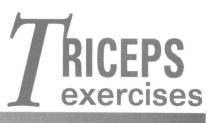

CABLE KICKBACK

Begin by standing in front of a low cable pulley apparatus with your body bent forward so that it is virtually parallel with the ground. Grasp a loop handle attached to the low pulley with your left hand and press your left arm against your side with your elbow bent at a 90-degree angle. With your palm facing your body, raise the handle by straightening your arm until it is parallel with the floor. Then, reverse direction and return the weight to the start position. After finishing the desired number of repetitions, repeat the process on your right.

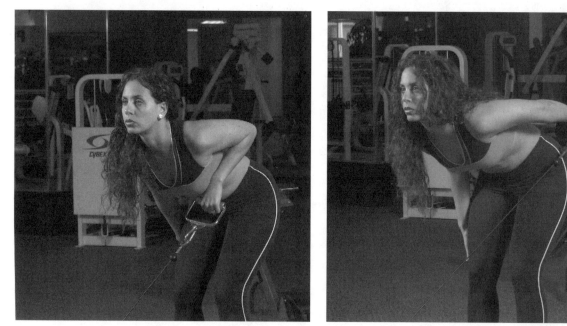

start   finish

For Home Use:
Attach a strength band to a stationary object and perform the move as described. ▶

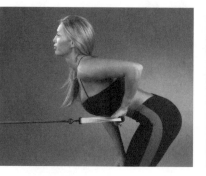 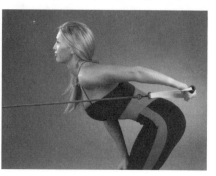

TRICEPS exercises

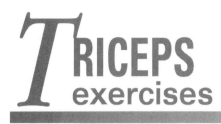
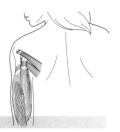

Group Three

Group Three exercises stress all heads of the triceps in roughly equal fashion. This is accomplished by performing movements where the upper arm is in a "mid-position," held out at a 90-degree angle to the torso. These exercises are great overall triceps builders, adding to the density of the muscle complex.

Performance of these moves requires total concentration to eliminate any ancillary shoulder involvement. Because the arms are held out in front of the body, there is a natural tendency to extend the shoulder joint as the weight is lifted. Avoid this inclination. Make sure that the upper arm remains at a 90-degree angle to the torso, moving only the forearm to complete each repetition.

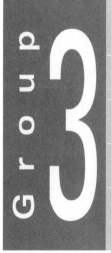

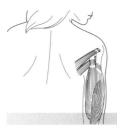
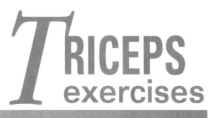
NOSEBREAKER

Begin by lying back on a flat bench with your feet planted firmly on the floor. Grasp an EZ-curl bar with your palms facing away from your body and straighten your arms so that the bar is directly over your chest (your arms should be perpendicular to your body). Keeping your elbows in and pointed toward the ceiling, slowly lower the bar until the weights are just above the level of your forehead. Press the bar back up until it reaches the start position.

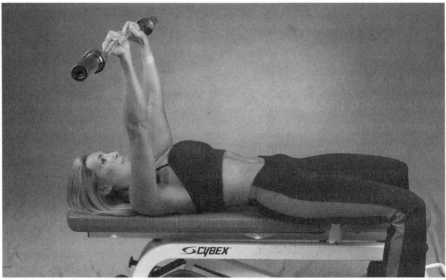

start

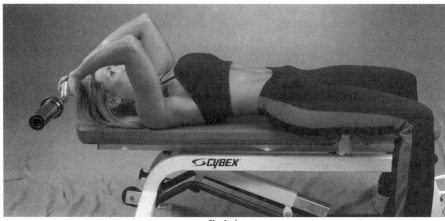

finish

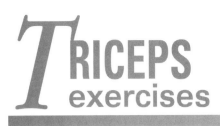

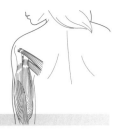

ONE-ARM DUMBBELL LYING TRICEPS EXTENSION

Begin by lying back on a flat bench with your feet planted firmly on the floor. Grasp a dumbbell with your right hand and straighten your right arm so that the dumbbell is directly over your chest (your right arm should be perpendicular to your body). Keeping your right elbow in and pointed toward the ceiling, slowly lower the dumbbell until it reaches a point just above the level of your forehead. Press the dumbbell back up until it reaches the start position. After performing the desired number of repetitions, repeat the process on your left.

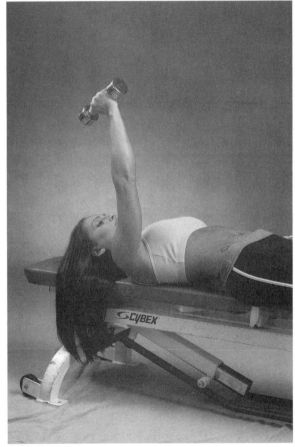

start

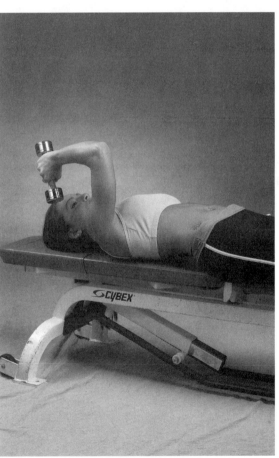

finish

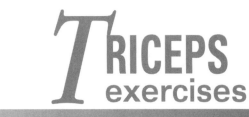

TWO-ARM DUMBBELL LYING TRICEPS EXTENSION

Begin by lying back on a flat bench with your feet planted firmly on the floor. Grasp a dumbbell in each hand and straighten your arms so that the dumbbells are directly over your chest (your arms should be perpendicular to your body). Keeping your elbows in and pointed toward the ceiling, slowly lower the dumbbells until they reach a point just above the level of your forehead. Press the dumbbells back up until they reach the start position.

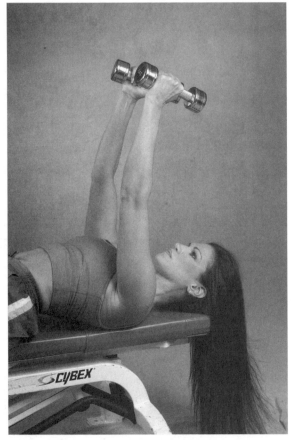

start

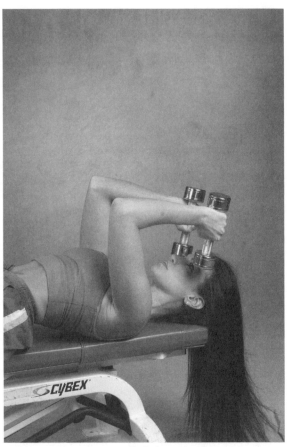

finish

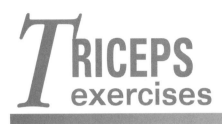

TRICEPS exercises

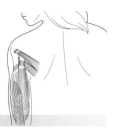

ONE-ARM STANDING CABLE TRICEPS EXTENSION

Begin by grasping a loop handle attached to a high cable pulley apparatus with your right hand and face away from the unit. Keep your elbow bent and your right arm at a position perpendicular to your body. Keeping your upper arm stable, straighten your right elbow until it is fully extended. Contract your triceps and then slowly lower the weight along the same path back to the start position. After performing the desired number of repetitions, repeat the process on your left.

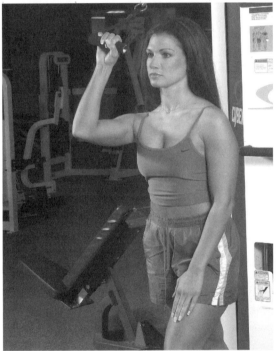

start

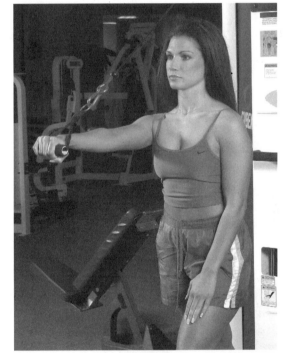

finish

For Home Use:
Attach a strength band to a stationary object and perform the move as described. ▶

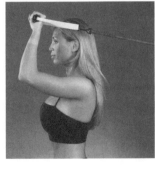

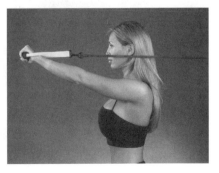

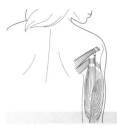 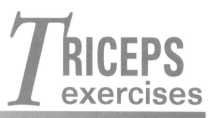

LYING CABLE TRICEPS EXTENSION

Begin by placing a flat bench in front of a low cable apparatus. Lie back on the flat bench and, with both hands, grasp a bar attached to the low pulley unit. Straighten your upper arms so that they are perpendicular to your body and allow your elbows to bend so that your forearms form a 90-degree angle to your upper arms. Keeping your upper arms stable, straighten your elbows until they are fully extended. Contract your triceps and then slowly lower the weight along the same path back to the start position.

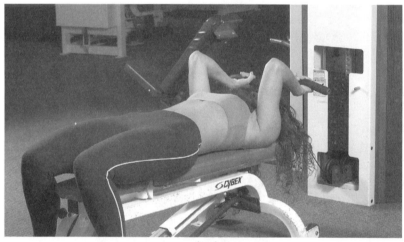

start

For Home Use:
Attach a strength band to a stationary object and perform the move as described. ▼

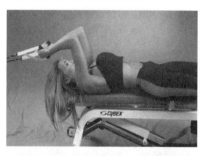

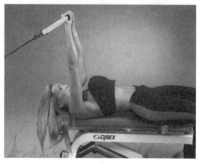

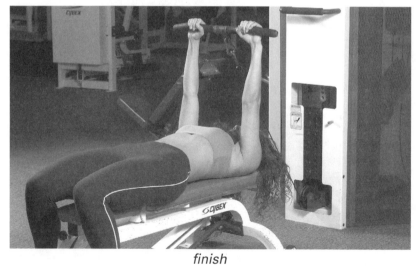

finish

Table 7.1 summarizes the exercises for Terrific Triceps.

TABLE 7.1

SUMMARY OF EXERCISES FOR TERRIFIC TRICEPS

Group One	Group Two	Group Three
One-Arm Overhead Dumbbell Extension	Rope Pressdown	Nosebreaker
Two-Arm Overhead Dumbbell Extension	Dumbbell Kickback	One-Arm Dumbbell Lying Triceps Extension
Seated Cable Overhead Extension	Triceps Bench Dip	Two-Arm Dumbbell Lying Triceps Extension
Standing Overhead Rope Extension	One-Arm Reverse Pressdown	One-Arm Standing Cable Triceps Extension
Seated Overhead EZ-Curl Extension	Cable Kickback	Lying Cable Triceps Extension

Sample Workouts

The following sample routines are provided for illustrative purposes. There are many other possibilities at your disposal, so be sure to experiment with different combinations.

Workout One

⇒ Two-Arm Overhead Dumbbell Extension

⇒ Cable Kickback

⇒ Nosebreaker

Workout Two

⇒ Seated Overhead EZ-Curl Extension

⇒ Bench Dip

⇒ One-Arm Standing Cable Triceps Extension

Workout Three

⇒ One-Arm Overhead Dumbbell Extension

⇒ One-Arm Reverse Pressdown

⇒ Lying Cable Triceps Extension

Workout Four

⇒ Standing Overhead Rope Extension

⇒ Rope Pressdown

⇒ Two-Arm Dumbbell Lying Triceps Extension

BEAUTIFUL BICEPS

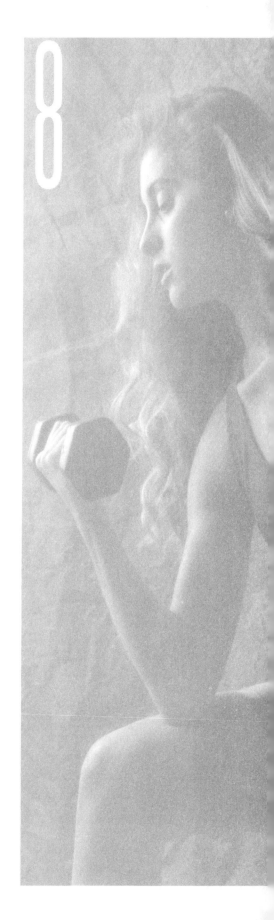

8

The biceps are the ultimate symbol of strength; no other part of the body is as glorified. After all, when someone asks you to make a muscle, it's the biceps that you flex, not your chest or thighs. And it's no wonder. The biceps are utilized in numerous activities of daily living. Whenever you lift, pull or carry an object, the biceps play a crucial role in the action. Even simple tasks such as opening a door or brushing your hair require the assistance of the biceps. But while these chores may help to achieve a basic level of muscular conditioning, the submaximal nature of the associated stimuli isn't enough to significantly improve muscle tone. The reality is, you're just not going to see much in the way of biceps development without targeted training.

Make no mistake, the biceps isn't all about strength and function; it's extremely important from an aesthetic standpoint, too. A lack of biceps development gives your upper extremities a sticklike appearance—effects that are magnified when you go sleeveless. Not only does this detract from the presentation of your arms, it can actually ruin the symmetry of your entire physique. Your torso seems blockier, your hips wider and your thighs thicker. In the absence of toned biceps, virtually every other muscle loses some impact.

Fortunately, with the right approach, the biceps is relatively quick to respond to exercise. It's one of the first places that you'll notice results from your training efforts. The reason is simple: There just isn't much fat to obscure it from view. While the triceps region tends to be an adipose storehouse, the area around the biceps is usually quite lean. Consequently, even small increases in muscular development really make the biceps stand out. Any time you flex your elbow, a muscle pops up for all to see!

The biceps shouldn't get all the glory here, though. Another muscle called the *brachialis* is equally important. The brachialis combines with the biceps to carry out any type of arm curling movement. The two muscles are synergistic, working in a complementary fashion. You can't use one without activating the other. Some studies have shown that the brachialis is even more powerful than the biceps, providing up to 70 percent of muscular strength during elbow flexion.

The brachialis also contributes to the aesthetic appeal of your upper arms. When properly developed, it augments the biceps and enhances upper extremity contour and detail. This gives your arms a full, rounded appearance, with better shape and breadth.

Realize, though, that because the biceps and brachialis are such small muscles, they can easily become overtrained. Smaller muscles generally have a reduced recovery ability (especially when they are predominantly fast-twitch) and therefore are more susceptible to this malady. In addition, assuming that you adhere to a well-structured total body training regimen (and hopefully you do), these muscles receive a great deal of ancillary stress almost every time you work out. Consequently, excessive targeted training can short-circuit the recuperation process, ultimately impairing muscular development.

In order to avoid this fate, pay strict attention to the effects of training on your biceps/brachialis. If they are continually sore or simply not responding to the demands of intense exercise, you might need to cut back on their training frequency. Past a certain point, additional training is superfluous and actually becomes counterproductive to the quest for shapely arms.

Anatomy of the Biceps/Brachialis Complex

The top portion of the upper arm is comprised of the biceps and brachialis. Let's take a look at the form and function of each muscle:

➡ The ***biceps brachii*** is a fusiform-shaped muscle that has two heads. The short head originates on the coracoid process of the anterior scapula (shoulder blade). The long head takes its origin from the supraglenoid tubercle of the scapula. Both heads attach to the radius (a small bone in the forearm). The biceps has two main functions: to flex (curl) the elbow and supinate the hand (turn the palm up towards the ceiling). Because the long head crosses the glenohumeral joint, it also has various roles in shoulder function—a fact that allows for additional bodysculpting capabilities.

⇢ The ***brachialis*** originates on the humerus (upper arm bone) and attaches on the coracoid process of the ulna (a small bone in the forearm). It has only one function: to flex the elbow.

Figure 8.1 provides an anatomical diagram that shows the location of the biceps and brachialis muscles.

FIGURE 8.1
Biceps and Brachialis Muscles

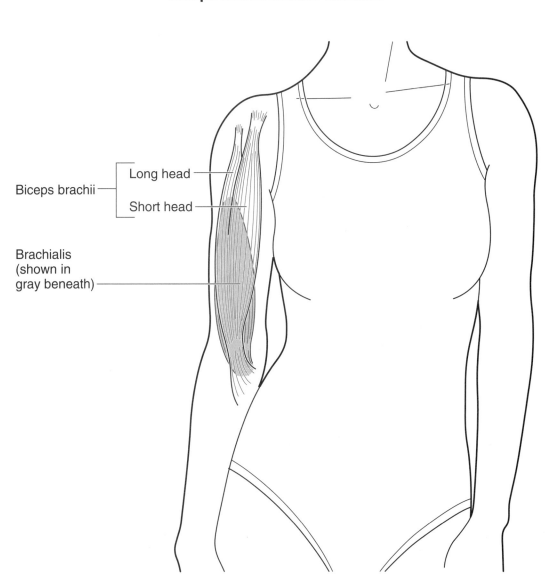

Biceps "Dos and Don'ts"

The following points should be kept in mind during biceps training.

➧ **Don't** *use your lower back when training your biceps.* One of the biggest mistakes made during biceps training is to perform "cheat curls," jerking the weight up by hyperextending the lower back. This is especially prevalent on the last few reps of a set, when training becomes increasingly difficult. However, while "cheat curls" will help you to get past a sticking point and complete a repetition, they place a great deal of stress on the lumbar region, making the lower back increasingly susceptible to injury.

➧ **Do** *keep your back tight throughout performance.* Your upper body should remain completely stationary, allowing your biceps to generate all the force to complete each rep.

➧ **Don't** *lock out your elbows when training your biceps.* All too frequently, women completely straighten their legs at the start of a rep. However, not only does this take stimulation away from the biceps muscles, it also places a great deal of stress directly on the joints.

➧ **Do** *stop just short of a lockout,* keeping continuous tension on your biceps at all times. There should be a slight bend in your elbows at the start position of each rep.

➧ **Don't** *bend your wrists when training your biceps.* Women generally have weak wrist muscles. Hence, when performing arm curls, their wrists don't have the strength to overcome the weight lifted. This causes the wrist to bend backward, placing increased stress on the area.

➧ **Do** *maintain rigidity in your wrist.* Consciously force the wrists to remain stable throughout each repetition. If necessary, add supplementary wrist exercises to develop strength in the area.

BICEPS exercises

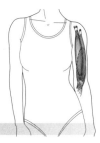

Group One

Group One exercises target the long head of the biceps. This is accomplished by performing movements where the upper arm is held at the sides or slightly behind the body (shoulder joint extension/hyperextension). Since the long head crosses the shoulder (glenohumeral) joint, it is somewhat stretched when the joint is extended and thereby generates increased force output during exercise.

The long head resides on the top, outer aspect of the upper arm. It has a lengthy tendon so that the diameter of its muscle belly is not as great as in the short head. However, because of its anatomical position, it is normally associated with the biceps "peak." Thus, increased development of this head will tend to promote the coveted "mountaintop" appearance of the biceps (although the actual shape of the peak is genetically predetermined and cannot be altered).

Your hands should always be supinated (palms turned up toward the ceiling) during these movements. Without supination, the biceps loses some of its force capacity. This decreases stress on the muscle, thereby diminishing muscular development.

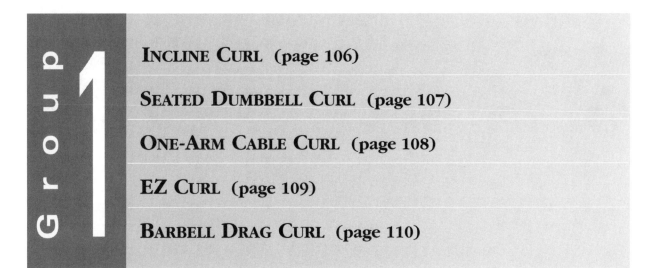

Group 1

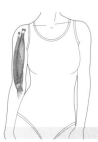

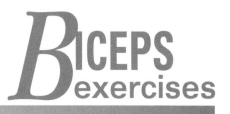

INCLINE CURL

Begin by lying back on a 45-degree incline bench. Grasp two dumbbells and allow the weights to hang by your hips with your palms facing forward. Keeping your upper arm stable, slowly curl the dumbbells upward toward your shoulders. Make sure your elbows stay back throughout the movement. Contract your biceps, then slowly return the weights to the start position.

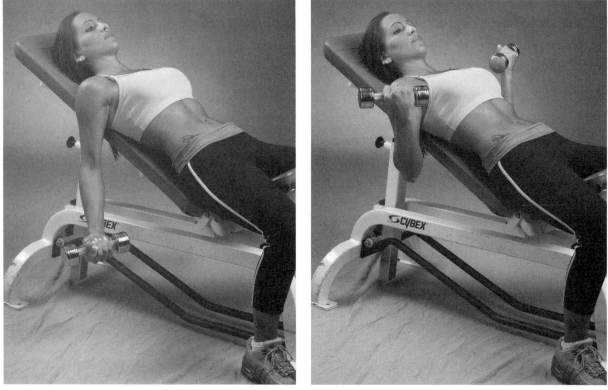

start   *finish*

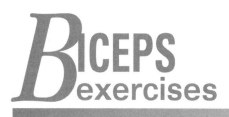 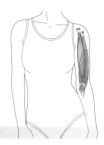

BICEPS exercises

SEATED DUMBBELL CURL

Begin by sitting at the edge of a flat bench. Grasp a pair of dumbbells and allow them to hang at your sides with your hands facing away from your body. Press your elbows into your sides and keep them stable throughout the move. Slowly curl the dumbbells up toward your shoulders and contract your biceps at the top of the move. Then, slowly reverse direction and return to the start position.

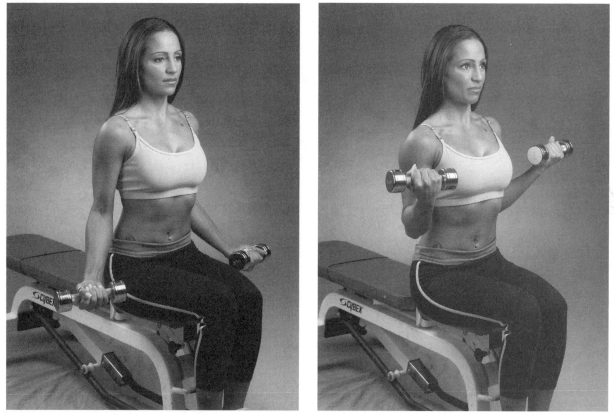

start   *finish*

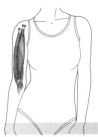

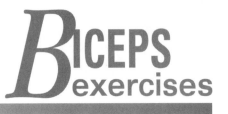
O**NE-ARM CABLE CURL**

Begin by grasping a loop handle attached to a low pulley apparatus with a palms-up, shoulder-width grip and face toward the machine. Maintain a slight bend to your knees. Press your left elbow into your sides and bring it behind your body as far as comfortably possible. Keeping your arm stable throughout the move, slowly curl the handle up toward your shoulders and contract your biceps at the top of the move. Then, slowly reverse direction and return to the start position. After completing the desired number of reps, repeat the process on your right.

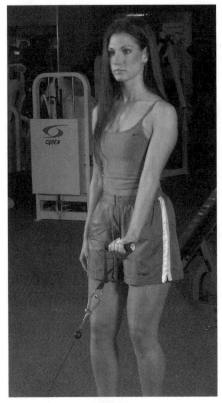

start

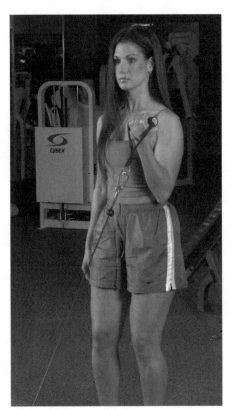

finish

For Home Use:
Attach a strength band to a stationary object and perform the move as described. ▼

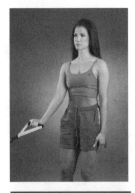

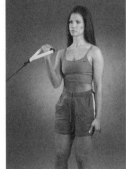

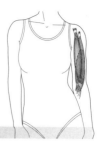

EZ CURL

Begin by grasping an EZ-curl bar with a palms-up, shoulder-width grip. Maintain a slight bend to your knees and press your elbows into your sides, keeping them stable throughout the move. Slowly curl the bar up toward your shoulders and contract your biceps at the top of the move. Then, slowly reverse direction and return to the start position.

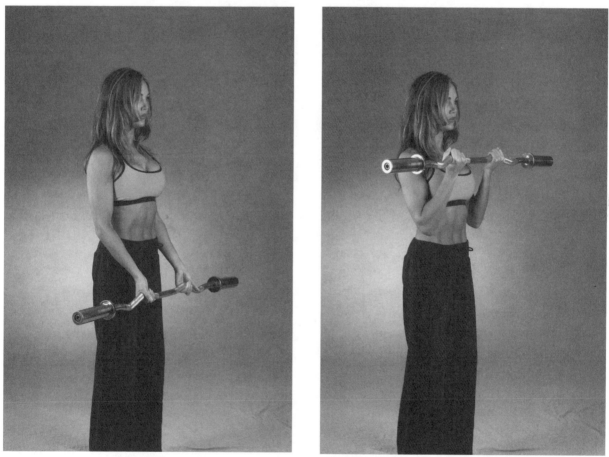

start   *finish*

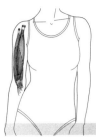
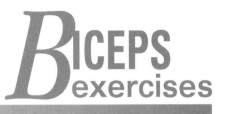

BARBELL DRAG CURL

Begin by grasping a barbell with a palms-up, shoulder-width grip. Maintain a slight bend to your knees. Press your elbows into your sides and bring them behind your body as far as comfortably possible. Keeping your upper arms stable throughout the move, slowly curl the bar up toward your shoulders and contract your biceps at the finish position. Then, slowly reverse direction and return to the start position.

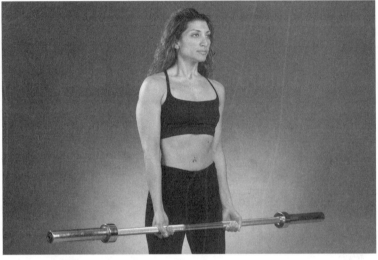

start

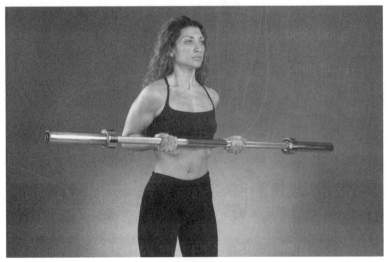

finish

BICEPS exercises

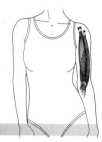

Group Two

Group Two exercises target the brachialis. This is accomplished by keeping your hands in a neutral position (palms facing toward the body) throughout the course of movement. These exercises really help to provide a polished look to the upper arms, creating delineation between the biceps and triceps.

Certainly, the biceps will still be active during these moves. But one of the functions of the biceps is to supinate the hand (turn the hand so that the palm faces up toward the ceiling). If the arm is flexed without supination, the biceps can't exert optimal force. Conversely, since the brachialis is a pure arm flexor with no function at the hands, it assumes the dominant role during performance in the absence of supination.

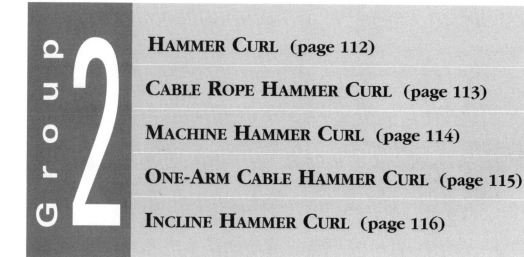

Group 2

HAMMER CURL (page 112)

CABLE ROPE HAMMER CURL (page 113)

MACHINE HAMMER CURL (page 114)

ONE-ARM CABLE HAMMER CURL (page 115)

INCLINE HAMMER CURL (page 116)

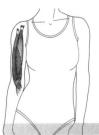

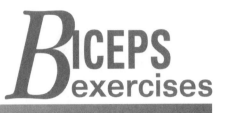

HAMMER CURL

Begin by grasping a pair of dumbbells and allow them to hang at your sides with your palms facing each other. Assume a comfortable stance with a slight bend to your knees and press your elbows into your sides, keeping them stable throughout the move. Slowly curl the dumbbells up toward your shoulders and contract your biceps at the top of the move. Then, slowly reverse direction and return to the start position.

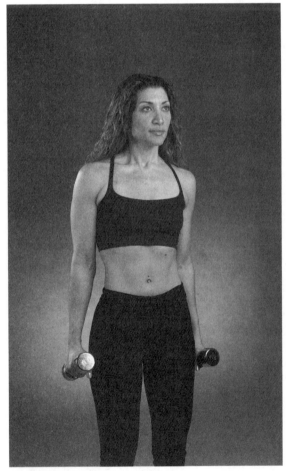

start

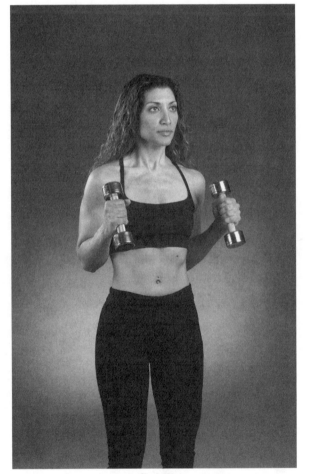

finish

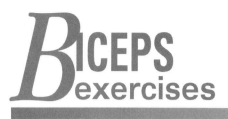

BICEPS exercises

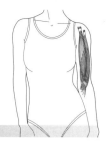

CABLE ROPE HAMMER CURL

Begin by grasping both ends of a rope that is attached to a low cable pulley. Bring your arms to your sides with your palms facing each other. Assume a comfortable stance with a slight bend to your knees and press your elbows into your sides, keeping them stable throughout the move. Slowly curl the rope up toward your shoulders and contract your biceps at the top of the move. Then, slowly reverse direction and return to the start position.

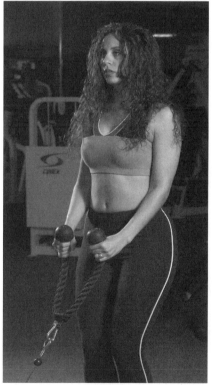

start

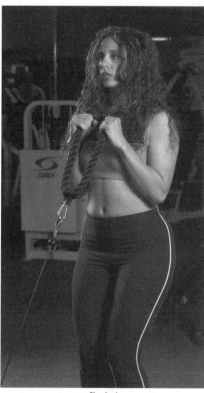

finish

For Home Use: Attach a strength band to a stationary object and perform the move as described. ▼

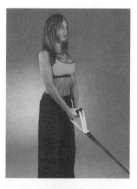

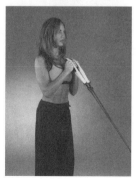

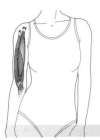
MACHINE HAMMER CURL

Begin by sitting in a hammer curl machine and grasp the handles of the unit. Place your elbows on the pads with your palms facing each other. Slowly curl the handles up toward your shoulders and contract your biceps at the top of the move. Then, slowly reverse direction and return to the start position.

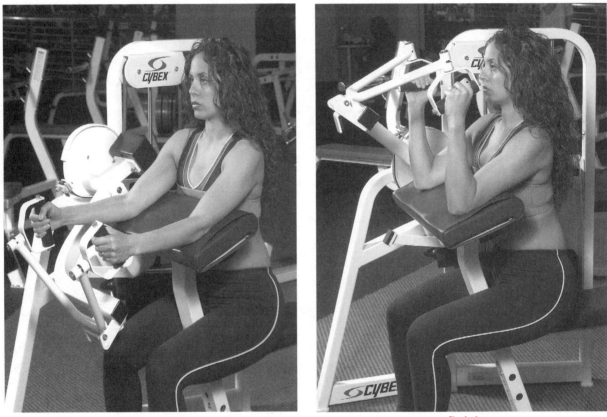

start   *finish*

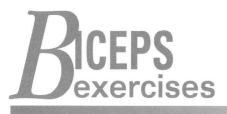

BICEPS exercises

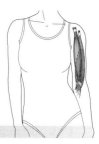

ONE-ARM CABLE HAMMER CURL

Begin by grasping the end of a rope that is attached to a low cable pulley with your left hand. Bring your left arm to your side with your left palm facing your torso. Assume a comfortable stance with a slight bend to your knees and keep your left upper arm stable throughout the move. Slowly curl the rope up toward your shoulders and contract your left biceps at the top of the move. Then, slowly reverse direction and return to the start position. After completing the desired number of reps, repeat the process on your right.

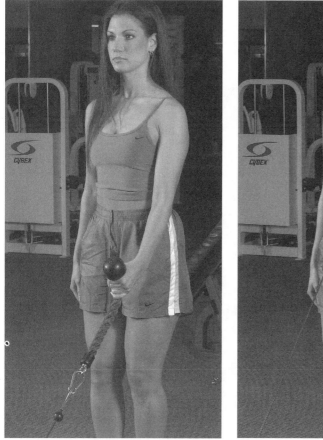

start

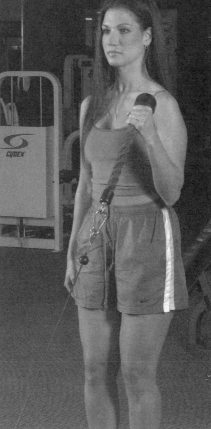

finish

For Home Use: Attach a strength band to a stationary object and perform the move as described. ▼

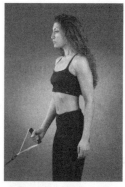

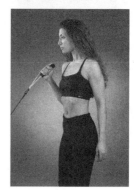

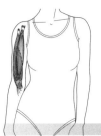

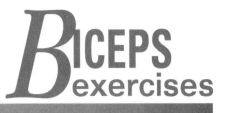

INCLINE HAMMER CURL

Begin by lying back on a 45-degree incline bench. Grasp two dumbbells and allow the weights to hang by your hips with your palms facing each other. Keeping your upper arms stable, slowly curl the dumbbells upward toward your shoulders. Make sure your elbows stay back throughout the movement. Contract your biceps, then slowly return the weights to the start position.

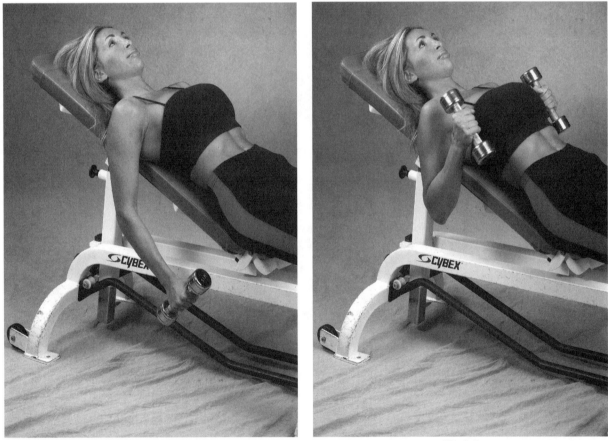

start   *fiinish*

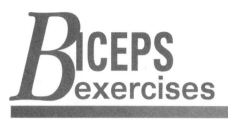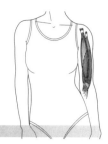

BICEPS
exercises

Group Three

Group Three exercises target the short head of the biceps. This is accomplished by performing movements where the upper arm is held out in front of the body (shoulder joint flexion) or to the sides (shoulder joint abduction). These exercises slacken the long head of the biceps, allowing the short head to exert maximal force.

The short head resides on the top, inner aspect of the upper arm. It is slightly larger in overall diameter than the long head and therefore contributes more toward the girth of the biceps. When fully developed, a split can be seen between the two biceps heads—a true sign of elite conditioning.

As with Group One exercises, the hands should always be supinated (palms turned up toward the ceiling) during performance. Without supination, the biceps loses some of its force capacity. This decreases stress on the muscle, thereby diminishing muscular development.

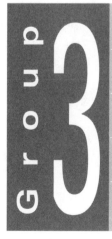

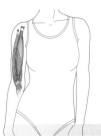

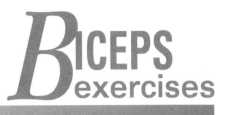

CONCENTRATION CURL

Begin by sitting at the edge of a flat bench with your legs wide apart. Grasp a dumbbell in your left hand and brace your left triceps on the inside of your left knee. Straighten your arm so that it hangs down near the floor. Slowly curl the weight up and in along the line of your body, contracting your biceps at the top of the move. Then, slowly reverse direction and return to the start position. After completing the desired number of reps, repeat the process on your right.

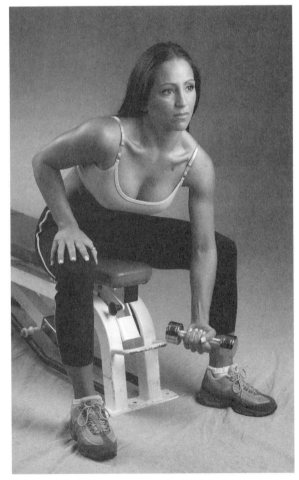

start

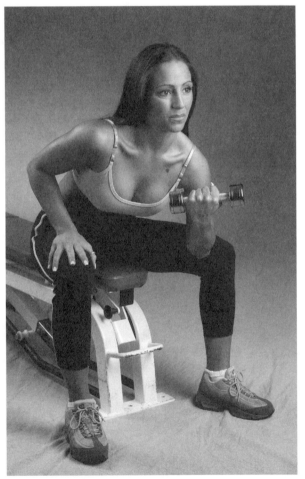

finish

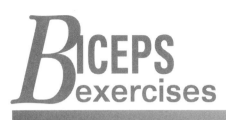
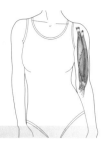

BICEPS exercises

PRONE INCLINE CURL

Begin by lying face-down on a 45-degree incline bench. Grasp two dumbbells and allow the weights to hang straight down from your shoulders with your palms facing away from your body. Slowly curl the dumbbells upward toward your shoulders, keeping your upper arms stable throughout the movement. Contract your biceps and then slowly return the weights to the start position.

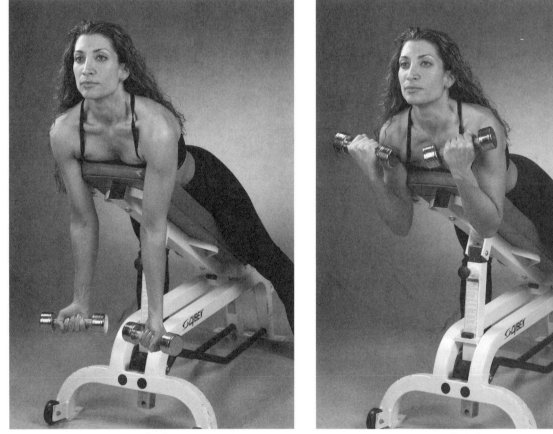

start   finish

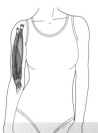

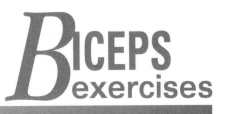

ONE-ARM DUMBBELL BENCH PREACHER CURL

Begin by grasping a dumbbell with your right hand. Place the upper portion of your right arm on an incline bench and allow your right forearm to extend just short of locking out the elbow. Keeping your upper arm pressed to the bench, slowly curl the dumbbell upward toward your shoulders. Contract your biceps and then slowly return the weights back to the start position. After completing the desired number of reps, repeat the process on your left.

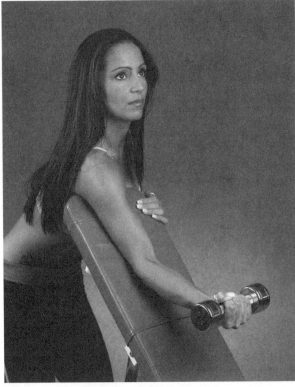

start

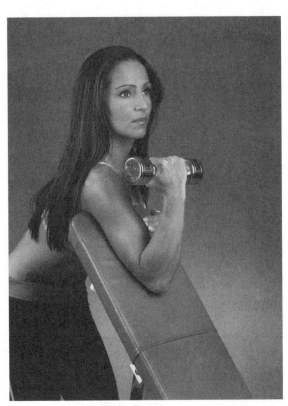

finish

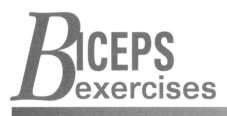

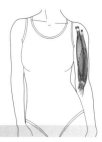

ONE-ARM CABLE PREACHER CURL

Begin by placing the upper portion of your right arm on an incline preacher bench. Grasp a loop handle attached to a cable pulley and allow your right forearm to extend just short of locking out the elbow. Keeping your upper arm pressed to the bench, slowly curl the loop handle upward toward your shoulders. Contract your biceps and then slowly return the weights to the start position. After completing the desired number of reps, repeat the process on your left.

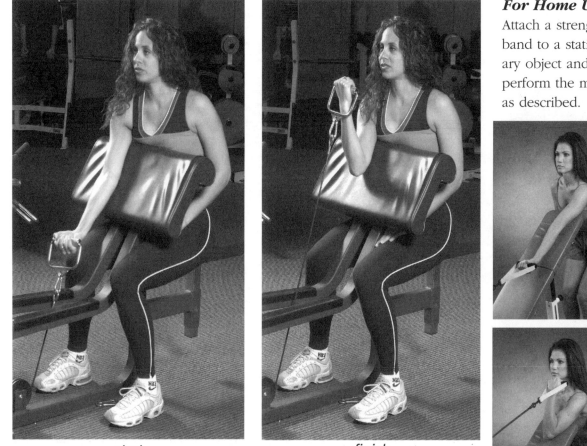

start

finish

For Home Use: Attach a strength band to a stationary object and perform the move as described. ▼

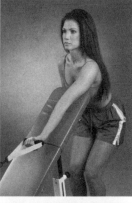

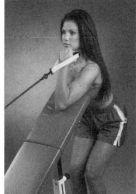

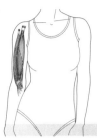 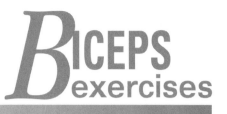

ONE-ARM HIGH CABLE CURL

Begin by grasping a loop handle attached to a cable pulley with your right arm. Allow your right arm to extend just short of locking out at the elbow so that it is parallel with the ground. Keeping your upper arm stable, slowly curl the loop handle upward toward your shoulders. Contract your biceps and then slowly return the weights to the start position. After completing the desired number of reps, repeat the process on your left.

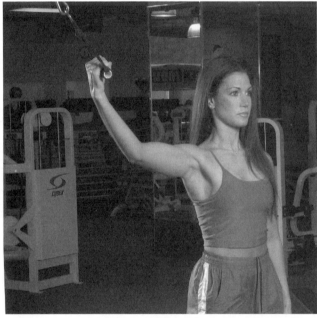 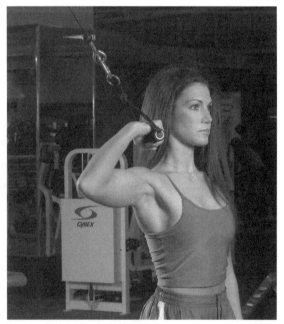

start   *finish*

For Home Use: Attach a strength band to a stationary object and perform the move as described. ▶

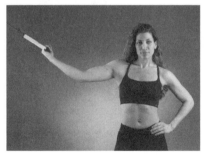 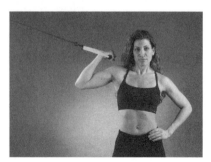

Table 8.1 summarizes the exercises for Beautiful Biceps.

TABLE 8.1

SUMMARY OF EXERCISES FOR BEAUTIFUL BICEPS

Group One	Group Two	Group Three
Incline Curl	Hammer Curl	Concentration Curl
Seated Dumbbell Curl	Cable Rope Hammer Curl	Prone Incline Curl
One-Arm Cable Curl	Machine Hammer Curl	One-Arm Dumbbell Bench Preacher Curl
EZ Curl	One-Arm Cable Hammer Curl	One-Arm Cable Preacher Curl
Barbell Drag Curl	Incline Hammer Curl	One-Arm High Cable Curl

Sample Workouts

The following sample routines are provided for illustrative purposes. There are many other possibilities at your disposal, so be sure to experiment with different combinations.

Workout One

➠ EZ Curl

➠ Machine Hammer Curl

➠ Concentration Curl

Workout Two

➠ Incline Curl

➠ One-Arm Cable Hammer Curl

➠ Prone Incline Curl

Workout Three

➠ One-Arm Cable Curl

➠ Cable Rope Hammer Curl

➠ One-Arm Dumbbell Bench Preacher Curl

Workout Four

➠ Seated Dumbbell Curl

➠ Hammer Curl

➠ One-Arm High Cable Curl

STOKING THE FAT-BURNING FURNACE

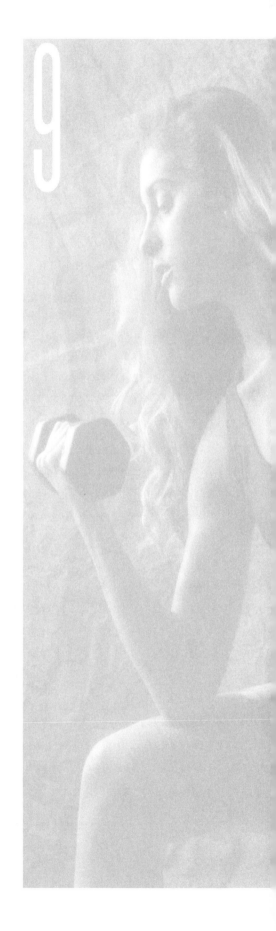

9

If you're like the great majority of women, you've probably done some type of aerobic training at some point in your life. There's a good chance you've even performed aerobics on a regular basis. Whether it's jogging, biking, kickboxing, or any of the other dozens of cardiovascular activities, women gravitate to aerobics like bees to honey.

Unfortunately, aerobics are often misunderstood. There is a prevailing misconception that aerobics are the key to physical perfection: Just get on the treadmill or take a few classes and you'll turn your body into a work of art. However, aerobics actually do little to improve your muscular shape and hardness. Without targeted bodysculpting, you'll never develop appreciable muscle tone and your body will end up loose and flabby—even if it's devoid of body fat.

Nevertheless, aerobics are an important component in a fitness regimen. Besides having a positive impact on your cardiovascular health, aerobics also play a significant role in body aesthetics. Let's take a look at these benefits:

➠ *Aerobics expedite fat burning.* A large portion of the calories that are expended during aerobic training are derived from fat. Depending on your exercise intensity, a single session of cardio can burn more than 20 grams of fat—enough to offset the amount in a greasy burger and fries. But the fat-burning effects extend beyond the immediate. Your metabolism remains elevated even after you have finished training, prolonging fat burning for up to several hours after your session. Moreover, your mitochondria (cellular furnaces where fat burning takes place) expand in size and number, and your aerobic enzymes (chemical messengers that accelerate the fat-burning process) increase in quantity. Over time, these factors allow your body to rely more on utilizing fat for fuel rather than glycogen (carbohydrates), helping to sustain long-term weight management.

➠ *Aerobics improve muscular endurance.* When you lift weights, your body converts glucose into the high-energy compound adenosine triphosphate (through a process called *glycolysis*) to fuel exercise performance. During this conversion process, lactic acid is produced and rapidly accumulates in your muscles as you train. When lactic acid builds up past a certain point, you experience an intense burning sensation in your muscles. Ultimately, the burn becomes so strong that it inhibits your ability to continue training. However, by increasing aerobic capacity, your cardiovascular system becomes more efficient at delivering oxygen to your working muscles. This helps to increase your lactate threshold—the point at which there is more lactic acid in your body than can be metabolized—and thereby delays the onset of lactic acid buildup. The end result is a greater capacity to train at a high level of intensity.

➠ *Aerobics enhance muscular recuperation.* Aerobics help to expand your network of capillaries—the tiny blood vessels that allow nutrients such as protein and carbohydrates to be absorbed into body tissues. The more capillaries that you have, the more efficient your body becomes in utilizing these nutrients for muscular repair. Capillaries also help to clear waste products, particularly carbon dioxide, from the food-burning process, further enhancing the efficiency of your nutrient delivery system. This accelerates the rate at which your muscles are able to get the resources needed for recuperation, helping to improve workouts and speed recovery.

Given these benefits, you would be remiss to exclude aerobics from your workout regimen. Aerobics provide the perfect complement to a strength-training routine, helping you attain a lean, hard appearance. But to get the most out of aerobics, you need to adhere to certain guidelines. There is a science to aerobics, and only by following established protocols will you optimize results.

Frequency

Because cardiovascular exercise is endurance oriented, many women believe it can be performed on a daily basis. However, while it's true that your body can tolerate a greater volume of aerobic exercise (as opposed to anaerobic activity), too much of it eventually will set back your progress and have a negative impact on your physique. Only by striking the right balance between exercise and rest will you reap maximal rewards.

During the recovery period, your body is able to regenerate its glycogen reserves. Glycogen is your body's primary energy source, giving you the strength and endurance to perform physical activities. Since cardio burns glycogen (as well as fat) during exercise performance, these reserves eventually become depleted, leaving you fatigued. Ultimately, your training ability is hampered, diminishing the quality of your workouts.

In extreme cases, performing an excess of aerobics can result in a condition called *overtraining syndrome* (OTS). Overtraining makes your body less efficient in utilizing fat for fuel and is apt to cannibalize your muscle tissue (due to a secretion of stress hormones) for energy. Moreover, it can throw off your biochemical balance, causing a variety of complications that include cessation of your period (amenorrhea), chronic fatigue, and other anomalies. To avoid this fate, you must constantly monitor your physical state, paying keen attention to the symptoms relating to overtraining (see the accompanying box). There is a fine line between training and overtraining; make sure you don't cross it.

SYMPTOMS OF OVERTRAINING

Overtraining syndrome (OTS) is a common exercise-related affliction. Studies show that it affects as much as 10 percent of all people who exercise on a regular basis. Due to a lack of understanding about the subject, OTS often ends up going undiagnosed.

The following are some of the symptoms relating to overtraining. If you experience two or more of these symptoms, you might be overtrained. If symptoms persist, get plenty of sleep and don't resume training until you feel mentally and physically ready.

- ▶ *Increased resting heart rate*
- ▶ *Increased resting blood pressure*
- ▶ *Decreased exercise performance*
- ▶ *Decreased appetite*
- ▶ *Decreased desire to work out*
- ▶ *Increased incidence of injuries*
- ▶ *Increased incidence of infections and flu-like symptoms*
- ▶ *Increased irritability and depression*

Depending on your individual situation, cardiovascular should be performed three to five days a week. You should assess your need to lose body fat and adjust the frequency of your aerobic training accordingly. Just make sure you don't overdo it. Allow your body at least two full days a week of complete rest from exercise. This will help to enhance recovery and ensure adequate regeneration of your energy supplies. When in doubt, err on the side of caution. Remember, with respect to exercise, less can be more!

Duration

You don't need to perform lengthy aerobic sessions to reduce body fat. I have seen women stay on the treadmill for hours on end. They are so consumed with losing weight that cardiovascular exercise consumes a significant portion of their day. However, not only is this unnecessary, it actually can be counterproductive. As long as you train properly, optimal results are achieved in a modicum of time.

During the initial stages of training, you may only be able to endure a few minutes of cardio. If you aren't aerobically conditioned, oxygen will be in short supply and you'll get winded rather easily. Don't let this get you down. Endurance tends to build up very rapidly. Within a few weeks, you'll see major improvements in your stamina and, before long, cardio will be a breeze.

Once you have built up sufficient endurance, your aerobic sessions should last a minimum of about 20 minutes. It is believed to take approximately this long before fat is optimally released from cells and becomes available to be used as fuel. On the other hand, there are diminishing returns to performing cardio for extended periods of time. Lengthy, drawn-out aerobic sessions take a toll on your body and can easily lead to overtraining. Thus, to avoid any negative consequences, limit your sessions to no more than 45 minutes in length. By keeping the duration of your sessions between these prescribed boundaries, you'll maximize fat burning while mitigating any potential downside risk.

Intensity

Intensity is the key determinant in burning fat. There is a direct correlation between physical effort and caloric expenditure; the harder you work, the more calories you expend.

Some fitness professionals have perpetrated the myth that, for optimal fat burning, aerobics should be performed at a low level of intensity. This theory is predicated on the fact that a greater proportion of fat is burned during low-intensity exercise as opposed to exercise done at a higher level of intensity. However, the selective use of fat for fuel doesn't necessarily translate into a greater amount of fat loss. The loss of body fat is contingent on the total amount of fat calories burned—not the percentage of calories derived from fat—and, from this standpoint, high-intensity exercise invariably comes out ahead.

For example, if you burn 200 calories in a half hour by walking on the treadmill at a low level of intensity, approximately 60 percent of these calories will come from fat, giving you a net fat loss of 120 calories. On the other hand, exercising for the same amount of time at a high intensity will burn approximately 400 calories, with 160 of these calories coming from fat (even though the percentage of calories derived from fat is only 40 percent). Thus, if fat burning is your aim, performing cardiovascular exercise at a high level of intensity is clearly your best bet.

But how do you go about quantifying aerobic intensity? Commonly, women gauge their effort based on perspiration. The more they sweat, the harder they think they're working. However, while sweat often is associated with rigorous exercise, it actually is a poor indicator of intensity. When you exercise, sweat is brought on by an elevation of your body temperature. Your body regulates its temperature by activating your sweat glands, which then release water through your pores as a cooling mechanism. Hence, sweat is an indicator that your body temperature is rising, not necessarily that you are exercising at an intense level.

While there are many viable ways to gauge aerobic intensity, one of the easiest and most effective methods is by exercising in your target training zone. Your target training zone is based on a percentage of your age-related maximal heart rate. It can be determined by subtracting your age from 220 and then multiplying by the desired training intensity percentage. For example, if you are 20 years old and want to train at 80-percent intensity, your target heart rate would be 160 beats per minute (220 − 20 = 200 × .8 = 160).

As a rule, your target training zone should be somewhere between 50 and 85 percent of your maximal heart rate. Keep your pace stable, beginning with a brief warm-up and finishing with a light cool-down. Every few minutes, check your pulse to make sure that you are maintaining your target zone. If your cardiovascular conditioning is poor, start out on the low end of the spectrum and gradually increase your intensity in increments of approximately 5 percent per week. It may take a while before you are able to maintain a high-intensity level; just be patient and it will happen.

WHEN'S THE BEST TIME TO EXERCISE?

In theory, it is best to perform aerobics first thing in the morning, on an empty stomach. The absence of food brings about a reduction in circulating blood sugar, causing glucose levels to fall. With a diminished availability of glucose, your body tends to rely more on fat to fuel your workout. Thus, from a fat-burning perspective, a case can be made for doing your cardio as soon as you roll out of bed.

However, not everyone functions well first thing in the morning. If you're more of a night bird, chances are that you'll sleepwalk through a morning workout. You'll have trouble generating sufficient intensity during training, resulting in poor exercise performance.

What's more, there actually is some evidence that exercising after a meal burns more calories than exercising on an empty stomach. Although the exact reason has not been determined, it is theorized that an increase in futile energy cycles or the post-prandial thermic effect of food may be at least partly responsible. Consequently, it is debatable whether the potential for selective lipolysis (fat burning) is more important than increased caloric expenditure; there is good reason to believe it isn't.

Therefore, in reality, the best time to exercise is when you are at your best. If you are a morning person, go ahead and train early. But if you don't really get going until you've been awake for several hours, by all means train later in the day. In the final analysis, let your biorhythms determine when you should work out.

Modalities

Consumers are forever searching for the "ultimate" cardiovascular activity, one that will literally melt away fat. Equipment manufacturers play into this mania. They are continuously flooding the market with new products, each promising to be the "premier fat-burning machine."

However, despite the hype, physiology dictates that no single activity can maximize your ability to burn fat; there simply is no one *best* cardiovascular exercise. As you may recall, the human body readily adjusts to an external stimulus by becoming more proficient. Hence, when the same exercise is used on a repeated basis, adaptation takes place, ultimately leading to diminished returns.

Only by cross training between different modalities can you prevent adaptation and thereby expedite the loss of body fat. Cross training is best accomplished by choosing several different activities and alternating them from one workout to the next. Not only does this constantly keep your body "offguard," but it also helps to reduce the likelihood of a training-related injury. Since each modality uses different muscles in exercise performance, your bones, muscles, and joints aren't subjected to continual impact. Accordingly, there is less wear and tear on your body, saving your musculoskeletal system from overuse.

Generally speaking, you are better off performing individual aerobic modalities rather than participating in group-based classes. Without question, aerobic classes can be fun. They provide a festive atmosphere, with lively music and dance-oriented maneuvers. They also can be a great place to socialize and meet new people, adding to the experience. For those who are not internally motivated to exercise, these factors can provide an impetus to become more active.

However, group-oriented activities have several drawbacks. First, by catering to the masses, it is unlikely that a class will specifically target your own heart rate. Second, because of the extreme, unorthodox nature of the movements involved, the risk of sustaining an injury is much greater in a class setting. So if you're looking for optimal results, group classes really aren't the best way to go.

Alternatively, individual aerobic modalities provide you with the ability to train within your target zone. Therefore, you can customize a routine to meet your specific needs, maximizing your fat-burning potential. And since individual modalities are executed in a controlled fashion, they tend to be much safer to perform.

So which aerobic modalities should you employ? In general, it makes sense to choose exercises that you enjoy. Theoretically, if you relish an activity, you'll more likely keep up with your routine. However, try to keep an open mind and experiment with as many different activities as possible. The majority of exercise modalities allow you to read, watch television, and/or listen to music while you train. These diversions can make even the most mundane activity seem tolerable. Remember, variety is the spice of exercise—keep an open mind.

THE Q-ANGLE

Due to an increased Q-angle (the angle formed between the knee and hip), women are predisposed to knee-related injuries. Since women tend to have naturally wide hips (to accommodate the demands of childbirth), they generally have a larger Q-angle than their male counterparts. A large Q-angle causes lateral displacement of the femur (thighbone), heightening patellar forces during impact activities. As a rule, the wider your hips, the greater the risk of injury.

Although a regimented strength-training program will help to improve knee stability, care should be taken to ensure proper safety. Repeated use of high-impact maneuvers should be avoided. If clinically indicated, a neoprene brace can be utilized to provide greater stabilization to the area.

Below is an overview of the five most popular pieces of aerobic equipment. These machines can be found in virtually any gym and also are available to purchase for home use. It is important to note, however, that the equipment quality can vary significantly. If you choose to buy, make sure to shop around and try out a number of different units.

➠ *Treadmill:* The treadmill is probably the most widespread aerobic apparatus. It can be used to walk, jog, or run—or any combination of the three. The more expensive units have such features as preprogrammed workouts, built-in heart rate monitors, adjustable inclines, and others.

There are those who eschew the treadmill, preferring to run in the park or the street. Exercising in the great outdoors allows you to get some fresh air and sunshine and provides a sense of being in touch with nature. These are powerful allures for making aerobics more enjoyable.

However, the potential hazards of outdoor running can outweigh the benefits. When you run, a tremendous amount of downward force is exerted on your lower extremities. Each stride results in joint compression forces of up to 33 times bodyweight. For example, a 130-pound woman can conceivably put more than 4,200 pounds of downward pressure on her joints each time her heel strikes the ground! Wet leaves, potholes, and other obstacles exacerbate the associated risks. This is why 70 percent of those who run on a frequent basis experience an injury to their lower extremities.

The treadmill helps to mitigate these dangers. Since a treadmill has a cushioned surface, it absorbs some of the impact to your shins and knees. Consequently, the risk of injury to your lower extremities is significantly reduced.

HAND WEIGHTS AND THE TREADMILL

By holding onto hand weights while walking, you can substantially increase the number of calories expended. This is an excellent way to burn additional fat while alleviating the wear and tear to the lower extremities. In fact, walking at 4 miles per hour with hand weights burns the same amount of calories as running at 5 miles per hour, with a 50-percent decrease in compression forces!

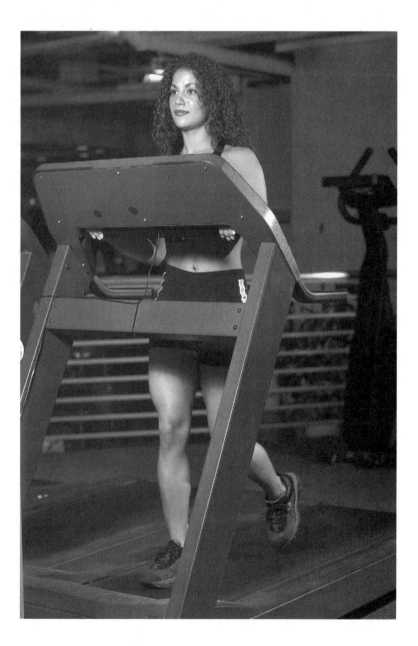

➠ ***Stationary Bike:*** Along with the treadmill, the stationary bike is an aerobic favorite. There are two basic types of bikes: upright and recumbent. Of the two, the recumbent is the decidedly better choice. It has an ergonomically designed seat that provides support for your back. This reduces stress to the lower lumbar region. The upright bike, on the other hand, has no such support. Hence, there is a tendency to lean forward during exercise, which can increase the potential for lower back injury.

Before using a bike, make sure to adjust the seat so that it corresponds to your height. Ideally, there should be a slight bend to your knees when pedals are at their lowest position. If your knees lock out, damage can occur to your connective tissue. Conversely, too much of a bend tends to overstretch the joint, which can also lead to injury.

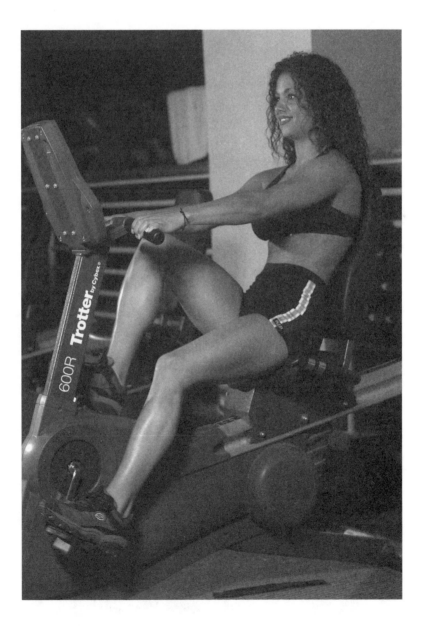

➠ ***Stair Climber:*** The stair climber (also called a *stair stepper*) is a mechanical version of, well, you guessed it, climbing stairs. Large pedals move in an up-and-down fashion, simulating the stair-climbing motion. When proper intensity is utilized, this can provide a terrific cardiovascular workout.

Unfortunately, some women avoid the stair climber, believing that it increases the size of their butt. Rest assured, nothing can be further from the truth. The fact is, it's virtually impossible to increase muscle mass significantly through the performance of *any* endurance-related cardiovascular activity. The reason for this is simple: Aerobic exercise relies predominantly on slow-twitch muscle fibers during performance, with little activation of fast-twitch fibers. If you remember, fast-twitch fibers are the only type of fibers that have the ability to increase in size substantially. Since the stair climber is aerobic in nature and therefore doesn't sufficiently activate fast-twitch fibers, it stands to reason that it can't contribute to building a substantial amount of muscle tissue in any part of the body, including your butt.

During performance, it is important to keep an upright posture; don't lean forward while stepping. Doing so places an inordinate amount of stress on the lumbar area, which easily can lead to lower back pain. Rather, maintain a slight lordotic curve (arched lower back), keeping your head up and chest out.

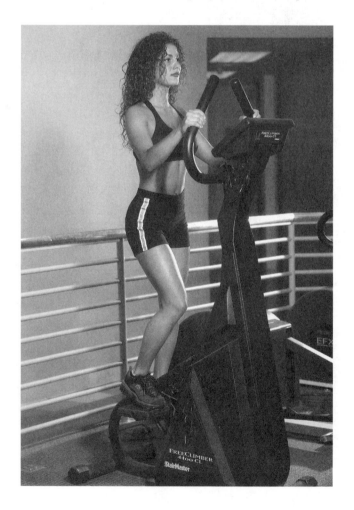

➡ ***Elliptical Trainer:*** The elliptical trainer is fast becoming a favorite in many gyms. Its sleek, space-age design is an instant allure and its unique motion creates the feel of "moonwalking."

From a practical standpoint, the main advantage of the elliptical trainer is that it tends to reduce stress to the lower extremities. Its fluid, nonimpact motion tends to be easier on the joints, which can be particularly beneficial for those who have existing injuries to the hips, knees or ankles.

During performance, you have the choice of pedaling in either a forward or backward direction. It is best to employ both options. This allows different muscle fibers to be recruited, providing more complete aerobic conditioning.

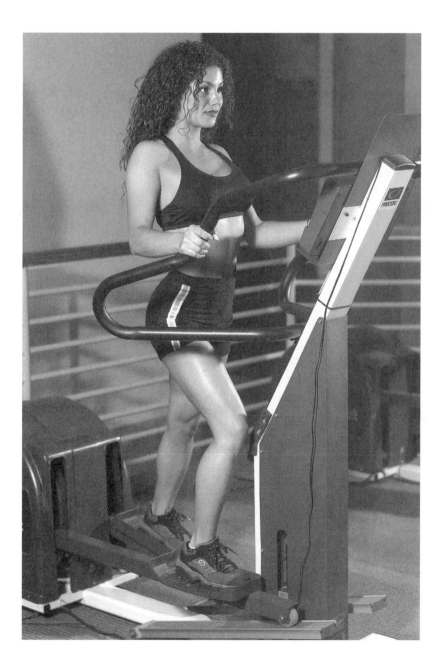

➡ ***Rowing Machine:*** The rowing machine is perhaps the most underutilized of all the cardiovascular modalities. With all the new aerobic devices on the market, the rowing machine basically has been relegated to second-tier status. Yet rowing is one of the best ways to condition the upper body—something lacking in most aerobic activities.

Contrary to popular belief, upper body aerobics promote a greater caloric expenditure when compared with activities that are limited to the lower body. This is largely attributable to the metabolic cost of stabilizer muscles that are recruited to support the torso when the arms are aerobically trained. Hence, aerobic exercise that involves the upper body actually is a very efficient means for expediting the loss of body fat. What's more, since cardiovascular benefits are specific to the muscles being worked, additional aerobic pathways (i.e., enzymes, mitochondria, capillaries, etc.) are established in the upper body, helping to expedite fat burning.

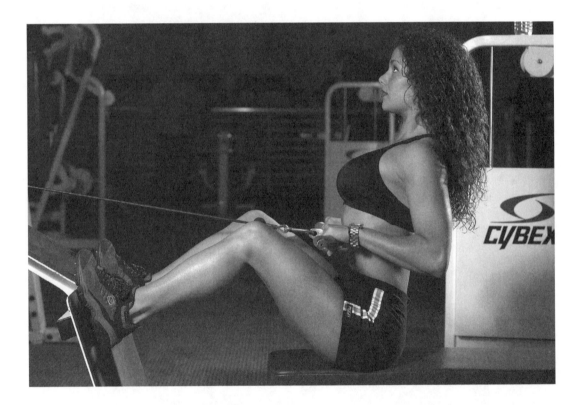

It must be noted, however, that upper body aerobics tend to elevate blood pressure during training. Because the circulatory capacity is lower in the arms than in the legs, there is an increased resistance to blood flow in this region, which, in turn, causes blood pressure to rise. Accordingly, for those with existing hypertension or cardiovascular disease, upper body aerobics may be contraindicated.

Also, it is probably best to perform upper body aerobics on days that you aren't training your arms. Since the arms are small muscles, they are easily fatigued. If you use these muscles in an endurance capacity, your strength levels during weight lifting will be impaired.

Of course, there are many other activities that make fine aerobic choices. Ballroom dancing, inline skating, cross country skiing—the list goes on and on. But regardless of which activities you choose to employ, make sure you are training with sufficient intensity to generate results. You'd need to play several hours of doubles tennis, for example, in order to burn the same number of calories as a half-hour run!

Table 9.1 summarizes the High-Energy Fitness™ protocols for cardiovascular training. As with weight training, proper manipulation of these protocols will determine how well you will ultimately excel in your efforts. Since your aerobic routine will impact on your weight-training program, striking the right balance between the two is essential in optimizing your physique. It is advisable to proceed cautiously here, starting with the minimum recommended levels and advancing with care. While the usual inclination is to go all out, you run the risk of pushing the envelope too far. As with most things in life, discretion is the better part of valor.

TABLE 9.1
HIGH-ENERGY FITNESS™ PROTOCOLS FOR CARDIOVASCULAR TRAINING

Duration	Frequency	Intensity	Modalities
20 to 45 minutes per session	3 to 5 days a week	50% to 85% of maximal heart rate, progressively increasing intensity over time	Alternate between as many different modalities as possible

EAT TO LOSE

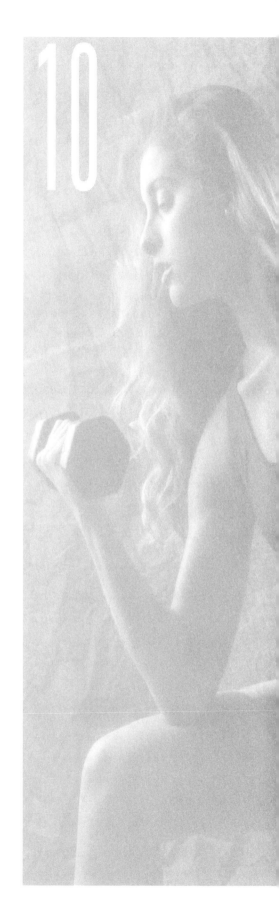

Virtually every woman is, at one time or another, on a diet. Slim is in, and women are willing to try almost anything in order to win the battle of the bulge. There are high-carb/low-fat diets, low-carb/high-fat diets, all-fruit diets, no-fruit diets, and even cabbage soup diets! From Atkins to the Zone, diets span the alphabet from A to Z.

However, the stark reality is that diets don't work! While most of these programs will induce temporary weight loss, they simply don't provide the ability to sustain this weight loss over the long haul. They are short-term solutions to a long-term problem and neglect to teach a woman proper eating patterns. Sadly, only 10 percent of those who go on a diet are able to keep the weight off after a year's time.

Worse yet, repeated cycles of weight loss and regain (called *yo-yo dieting*) can severely suppress metabolism and cause a rebound effect. During each diet cycle, the body continually trains itself to survive on fewer and fewer calories. Hence, it becomes increasingly more difficult to shed unwanted pounds and, in the end, regained weight is almost always higher than it was before dieting.

Actually, when applied to weight loss, the term *diet* is a misnomer. If you look in the dictionary, a diet is defined as "food and drink regularly provided or consumed." It is a normal meal plan that provides habitual nourishment, not a quick means to lose weight. Thus, from here on, the term *diet* will be used in the context of its intended meaning—to describe a regimented program of eating.

It is important to realize that there is no single "best" diet. Every woman has a unique nutritional profile and will respond differently to various foods based on a host of genetic and lifestyle factors. Things such as metabolic rate, insulin sensitivity, food allergies, and activity level all influence dietary requirements. Therefore, you can't simply follow a cookie-cutter nutritional prescription and expect it to work for you. Chances are, your specific needs won't be adequately addressed.

The key to promoting long-term, sustainable weight management is to develop a sound nutritional strategy that becomes a way of life. An effective program balances caloric intake with caloric expenditure, stabilizes insulin and increases metabolism. It must be sensible as well as practical. My approach to nutrition combines all of these facets. The program that I espouse is based on nutritional science, not gimmicks. It is specific in its recommendations, yet it is flexible enough to be adapted to your individual needs. Whether you want to lose, gain or maintain your current weight, this program will help you achieve your goals.

Before discussing which foods to eat, you need to determine your caloric intake. Calories *do* count and, despite the claims of some so-called nutritional "experts," the amount of food that you ingest will have a major impact on whether weight is gained or lost.

The first step in determining caloric intake is to figure out your daily caloric maintenance level (DCML): the number of calories required each day to maintain a stable body weight. A simple way to estimate DCML is to multiply your bodyweight by 12 (bodyweight ✕ 12). Thus, a woman who weighs 120 pounds would need approximately 1,440 calories to maintain her current weight. While this formula only provides a crude approximation of daily caloric intake, it at least gives you a starting point from which to work. From here, modifications can be made based on individual requirements.

If weight loss is desired, your DCML must be adjusted so you expend more calories than you consume. This is simple mathematics. You can eat all the "right" foods, but if you take in too many calories from these foods, weight gain is inevitable. For example, consuming as few as 100 extra calories a day—the amount found in a handful of nachos or a dozen French fries—can result in a yearly weight gain of more than 10 pounds! Only by creating a caloric deficit is weight loss possible.

For safe, effective weight loss, a maximum of 1 to 2 pounds can be lost per week. Don't be lured in by unscrupulous ads that promise to take off 30 pounds in 30 days. These quick-fix programs are unhealthy and counterproductive. When calories are severely restricted, up to 45 percent of the energy deficit is derived from burning muscle tissue for fuel. This can account for as much as 1 pound a week of muscle loss. As previously discussed, muscle is highly metabolic. It speeds up resting metabolic rate and thereby accelerates the body's ability to burn fat. Thus, by depleting muscle tissue, fat-burning is inhibited, inevitably leading to an increase in body fat.

Your best bet is to take it slow. A loss of 1 pound per week might not seem like a lot on the surface but, over the course of a year, it equates to a 50-pound drop. Start out with a 300-calorie reduction in your DCML and then gradually increase this amount if necessary. But don't go overboard—remember, rapid weight loss will sabotage your long-term fitness goals. If you experience a loss of more than 2 pounds in a week, increase caloric intake accordingly to stay in the prescribed range.

Initially, it can be helpful to weigh your food on a scale. A digital food scale is relatively inexpensive and easy to use. While this may seem like a chore, it really is worth the effort. Weighing your food takes only a few seconds and requires no cleanup. Within a short period of time, you'll develop a sense of how much to eat and soon will be able to estimate portion sizes on your own.

Once you have determined your caloric intake, you must now focus on the percentage of calories that will be derived from carbohydrates, protein and fat—the so-called "macronutrients." To get the most out of your diet, it is imperative that you take in the right mix of these nutrients. Those who believe the old adage that "a calorie is a calorie" are sadly mistaken. Each nutrient has specific functions and affects the body in different ways. Let's discuss how these nutrients should be apportioned for optimal benefits.

Carbohydrates

For those who are trying to stay lean, carbs can be a double-edged sword. On one hand, carbs are the body's preferred source of metabolic energy. They help to preserve tissue proteins, assist in fat metabolism and stoke the central nervous system.

Carbs are particularly important as you exercise. The compounds derived from carbohydrate breakdown are stored as glycogen in your muscles and liver. Glycogen is the primary fuel used to power your muscles during intense workouts. It provides an instant source of energy that can be accessed on demand, enabling you to train in an all-out fashion.

When carbohydrates are severely restricted in the diet, your body has to convert amino acids into glucose (through a process called *gluconeogenesis*) in order to meet short-term energy needs. However, this conversion process is very inefficient and fails to supply adequate energy reserves. Ultimately, your stamina begins to wane and you soon become lethargic and irritable. Complications including nausea, headaches and dizziness are apt to occur. There is a degradation in exercise performance, diminishing your capacity to generate lean muscle tone. Overall, your ability to function at a high level is seriously impaired.

On the other hand, carbs trigger the release of insulin in the body. When ingested, carbs are broken down into simple sugars. In turn, the pancreas must secrete insulin to clear the surplus sugar from the bloodstream. However, while insulin plays an important role in regulating body function, it also can be detrimental to weight management. You see, insulin is a storage hormone that is directly responsible for converting sugars into fat as well as inhibiting the conversion of stored fat into energy. This double whammy greatly increases the potential for body-fat storage.

Because of this effect on insulin, it is essential to regulate the types and amount of carbohydrates for optimal weight management. Make no mistake: All carbs are not created equal! Although most people know that it's important to cut back on fatty foods, they often are oblivious to the types of carbohydrates in their diet.

A common way to distinguish carbs is by their complexity. You've probably heard about the differences between "simple" and "complex" carbs. However, a better mode of classification is based on the glycemic index. The glycemic index provides a more accurate indication of how carbs affect insulin secretion. Carbs that cause a rapid elevation of blood sugar (glucose) are termed *high-glycemic,* while those that are "time released" and maintain stable levels of blood sugar are called *low-glycemic.*

High-glycemic carbs tend to have a negative impact on your physique. The problem with these foods is that they are rapidly assimilated, causing a spike in your blood-sugar levels. Consequently, a large quantity of insulin is needed to stabilize blood sugar. This increased insulin production turns on fat-storage mechanisms and blocks certain enzymes that are responsible for lipolysis (fat breakdown). Ultimately, excess nutrients are shuttled into adipose cells, resulting in a corresponding increase in body fat.

Furthermore, this rush of insulin clears sugars from your circulatory system in such an expeditious fashion that it creates a rebound effect, producing a sudden and dramatic drop in blood-sugar levels. A hypoglycemic state is induced, causing severe hunger pangs and food cravings. This creates a vicious cycle that encourages you to binge out on high-glycemic foods. As a result, more calories are consumed and fat storage is heightened even further.

Conversely, low-glycemic foods are broken down more slowly. They enter the bloodstream in a time-released fashion, keeping blood-sugar levels in check. Insulin, therefore, is released gradually into your system. Stable insulin levels mean reduced body-fat storage. And, because there's a steady stream of glucose, your energy levels remain high.

Hence, if you want to stay lean, keep your consumption of high-glycemic foods—especially refined sugars—to an absolute minimum. When eaten in abundance, they can be one of the biggest obstacles to maintaining a lean physique, perhaps even more so than foods laden with fat. Remember: Just because a food is "fat free" doesn't mean it won't make you fat—it also must be low glycemic to qualify as a healthy choice. Accordingly, stay away from such high-glycemic choices as sweetened cereals, potatoes, white rice, and white flour breads. Instead, replace them with oatmeal, yams, brown rice, and whole grains. If you do choose to consume a high-glycemic food, make sure you eat it in conjunction with a protein-based source. This will help to slow down absorption and mitigate its effect on insulin secretions.

Fiber is another important component of carbohydrate intake. There is a large body of scientific evidence indicating that a diet high in fiber is beneficial to your health. At the very least, fiber helps to maintain bowel regularity. Because fiber absorbs water in the large intestine, it causes your stools to become soft and fluffy, thereby preventing constipation. The increase in stool volume also helps to dilute the concentration of bile acids, which are thought to instigate the growth of malignant tumors. Studies have shown up to a 30-percent reduction in these malignancies with increased fiber intake, making fiber a potent cancer-fighting agent.

In addition, fiber consumption can cause a substantial decline in serum cholesterol levels. Reductions of up to 13 percent have been reported, with favorable effects on the ratio of "good" to "bad" cholesterol (HDL to LDL). Since each 1-percent drop in cholesterol translates into a 2-percent drop in the risk of developing heart disease, the cardioprotective effects of fiber are far-reaching.

Besides having a positive effect on your well-being, fiber also plays an important role in weight management. By forming a "gel" in the intestines, it inhibits the digestion and absorption of nutrients. As food passes through your intestines, some of the nutrients get trapped in the gel and end up being excreted before they can be metabolized. Hence, you can eat more food without having it stored in your system. In fact, it has been reported that, by simply doubling fiber intake from 18 to 36 grams, you reduce the available calories in your diet by more than 100 calories per day!

Fiber is found in a wide array of carb-based foods. Appendix A shows some of the more popular high-fiber foods as well as their corresponding fiber content. Consume them readily. By maintaining a high-fiber diet, you'll go a long way toward improving your health as well as your body.

Recommended Intake: Carbs should comprise approximately 40 to 50 percent of the calories in your diet. This will sufficiently replenish glycogen reserves without having an adverse effect on insulin levels. Start out on the low end of the spectrum, keeping carbs at the suggested minimum. If you feel lethargic or fatigued, increase carbs another 5 percent. If you still don't have enough energy, take carbs up to the maximum.

Green vegetables should make up a healthy portion of carb intake. On a volume basis, they are extremely low in calories and high in nutritional value. Think of them as green water—they can be consumed in large amounts without making you fat. A pound of broccoli, for instance, contains only about 120 calories (compare that to a pound of pasta, which has about 1,600 calories). Moreover, because of their bulk, green vegetables take up a large amount of space in the stomach. This helps to suppress food cravings, thereby preventing the urge to overeat. And considering that they are replete with vitamins and minerals, green vegetables should be a staple in your diet.

Protein

Without question, protein is the king of all nutrients. It provides the building blocks for enzymes and hormones, enables nerve and brain cells to communicate effectively with one another, and fosters the repair and growth of muscle tissue. Every cell in your body contains protein; life could not go on without it.

A diet high in protein has a multitude of benefits. First, protein has a greater thermic effect than any other nutrient. Because of its chemical structure, a great deal of energy is expended in the breakdown of protein. Up to 25 percent of protein-based calories are burned in this process. Of course, with fewer calories available for storage, the potential for weight gain is diminished.

Protein also is the most satisfying of all the macronutrients. On a calorie-for-calorie basis, protein fills you up more than either carbs or fat. This is largely due to the secretion of satiety hormones, especially cholecystokinin (CCK). Studies have shown that when people consume a calorie-restricted diet consisting of carbs, protein or fat, only those on the protein diet demonstrate a significant reduction in hunger sensation. Similar findings have been shown for caloric intake; people following a protein-based diet tend to eat significantly fewer calories than those on a carb- or fat-based diet. The evidence is clear: When protein consumption is high, you're less inclined to binge out on large meals.

In addition, adequate protein is necessary to remain in positive nitrogen balance, a condition that prevents the breakdown of muscle tissue and accelerates recuperation from exercise. When protein intake is insufficient, nitrogen is excreted at a greater rate than it's consumed, sending your body into a catabolic state. Overtraining is likely to occur and muscular development suffers.

Furthermore, as opposed to carbohydrates, protein has a negligible effect on insulin levels. Protein is not directly broken down into glucose. It must first undergo a complex conversion process called *deamination* before it can be assimilated and synthesized by the body. This helps to keep blood sugar in check, preventing the oversecretion of insulin. Moreover, protein tends to increase the production of glucagon, a hormone that opposes the effect of insulin. Since a primary function of glucagon is to signal the body to burn fat for fuel, fat loss, rather than fat gain, is promoted.

There is a widespread fallacy that high-protein diets are harmful to your health. This myth is based on the contention that a surplus of protein has a detrimental effect on kidney function. Undeniably, the digestion of protein results in the accretion of urea, a byproduct of amino acid breakdown. In theory, a large buildup of urea overtaxes the kidneys and impairs their ability to function. However, as long as you don't have existing renal disease, your kidneys are more than able to handle this overload. Provided you take in a sufficient quantity of fluids, any excess urea will be readily excreted from your body with no ill effect on renal function.

Recommended Intake: Protein should account for 30 to 40 percent of total calories, equating to roughly 1 to 1.25 grams of protein per pound of bodyweight. Hence, a woman weighing 120 pounds needs to consume a minimum of 120 grams of protein per day. Any less and you risk falling into a negative nitrogen balance. Disregard the United States Department of Agriculture (USDA) recommended daily allowance (RDA) for protein (an absurdly low .4 grams per pound of bodyweight). The RDA is based on the needs of sedentary people and doesn't take into account the increased demand required for active individuals.

Make sure that your choice of proteins comes from lean sources. Skinless poultry breast, lean red meats, seafood, and egg whites are excellent choices. For convenience, there are a wide variety of protein powders available at health stores and other outlets. Whey protein powders are generally your best choice, followed by egg, casein and vegetable sources.

Fat

Traditional wisdom has always been that if you want to maintain a lean physique, dietary fat should be kept to a bare minimum. For many years, the majority of sports nutritionists emphatically stated, "Eat fat and you'll get fat!" A legion of health-conscious consumers listened, and zero-fat diets soon became the rage. The prevailing sentiment was to cut out every last gram of fat from a diet. More recently, this view has softened, and certain classifications of fat are now being recommended as part of one's daily diet.

Certainly, fats are an essential nutrient and play a vital role in many bodily functions. They are involved in cushioning your internal organs for protection, aiding in the absorption of vitamins, and facilitating the production of cell membranes, hormones, and prostaglandins. Physiologically, it would be impossible to survive without the inclusion of fats in your diet.

Fats are classified into two basic categories: saturated and unsaturated. Saturated fats are abundant in many meats, oils and dairy products. They serve no biological purpose. After consumption, they either are stored in adipose cells throughout your body or become oxidized as fatty deposits in your arteries. Over time, your arteries narrow, resulting in severe atherosclerosis—a direct precursor to a heart attack. But that's not all. These fats tend to make your muscles less responsive to insulin and inhibit your body's ability to store sugars as glycogen. Studies have shown that the consumption of saturated fat is directly correlated with fat storage: The more you eat, the more you keep. Therefore, you must keep your consumption of saturated fats to an absolute minimum. Eliminate them at all costs.

Alternatively, unsaturated fats are healthier fats. In particular, specific types of unsaturated fats, called essential fatty acids (EFAs), are especially beneficial. EFAs cannot be manufactured by your body and hence, like vitamins, are an "essential" component in food. Due to their lack of saturation, they don't readily bond together (that's why they remain liquid at room temperature) and therefore can be synthesized for systemic use. In addition, they are extremely biologically active and help to increase your metabolic rate while enhancing the ability of your muscles to use insulin. Ultimately, this results in better fat metabolism and improved body composition.

The best sources of EFAs are found in soy products and deep-colored, cold-water fish such as salmon, mackerel and tuna. Flaxseed oil also contains high levels of EFAs. It comes in liquid form and either can be mixed into your foods or taken by the spoonful. Look for a brand that has a 3:1 ratio of omega-3 (linolenic acid) to omega-6 EFAs (linoleic acid).

TIPS FOR REDUCING SATURATED FATS

1. **Foods should be baked, broiled, steamed or microwaved. Never fry foods.**

2. **Prepare your foods "dry," without using lard, oil or butter in your cooking.**

3. **Trim all visible fat from your meats. Even lean cuts of meat normally have fat around the edges. Any fat that can be seen by the naked eye should be removed.**

4. **Remove the skin from poultry products. Do this *before* cooking since heat causes animal fat to seep into the meat.**

Recommended Intake: As a rule, limit your fat intake to no more than 20 percent of your total calories, with the majority coming from EFAs. Despite the recent prominence of high-fat diets, excess fat consumption will almost certainly have a negative long-term impact on your physique. Since virtually no energy is expended in their digestion, fats are more easily stored as body fat than any other nutrient. While proteins and carbs have a thermic effect on the body, the percentage of calories expended in the breakdown of fat is minimal.

Moreover, fats are calorically dense. Each gram of fat has nine calories, as compared to carbohydrates and protein, which have only four. Hence, a small portion of a fat-laden food has a much higher number of calories than a comparable portion of a low-fat food. For example, a sliver of chocolate cake might contain 200 calories, while it would take about 2 pounds of green beans to equal this amount. Since it takes a large quantity of fatty foods to sate the stomach, the potential for overeating is dramatically increased.

Thus, don't buy into the high-fat hype. Eat only enough to fulfill your basic requirements. If you want to look great sleeveless, lower fat is definitely the way to go.

Dining Out

Dining out is one of the greatest obstacles to dietary adherence. After all, it's fairly easy to eat properly when you're in the comfort of your own home. You can simply discard all the "bad" foods from your pantry or refrigerator, removing any temptation to binge on fattening foods. However, the average American eats away from home four days a week. Breakfast meetings, business lunches, dinner parties . . . dining out is an unavoidable fact of life.

Fortunately, with the proper approach, it's possible to maintain your nutritional regimen, even when you're away from home. By adhering to the following protocols, you can stay the course and maintain a terrific physique—regardless of where you may be dining.

➡ ***Hold the soup:*** As an appetizer, soup is king. Virtually every restaurant in the world has a "soup du jour." Soups are so popular that they're often included as a part of lunch and dinner specials. However, unbeknownst to many, soups are loaded with sodium. Not only does sodium elevate blood pressure levels, but it also causes your body to retain water. When too much sodium is ingested, fluid is drawn out of the cells and into the body's free spaces, resulting in a bloated appearance. Your feet and hands swell, your face becomes puffy and water accumulates beneath your skin—not a desirable condition for someone trying to stay lean. To avoid this fate, it's best to refrain from soups, choosing an alternate appetizer instead. In most cases, there are plenty of sodium-free options available. If not, skip the appetizer altogether; there's no rule that says you must have a multi-course meal.

➡ ***Skip the drinks:*** A healthy meal can be ruined by the inclusion of alcohol. Make no mistake; alcohol will make you fat. It is calorically dense, containing over seven calories per gram (as opposed to carbs and protein, which have four). Worse, many drinks are mixed with such high-calorie items as whole milk, soda and juice. For the most part, alcoholic beverages provide little or no nutritional value. They are "empty calories" that serve only to increase body-fat levels. Consequently, try to avoid alcohol at all costs. To quench your thirst, stick with water or club soda. If you must indulge, a white wine spritzer or lite beer is recommended.

➡ ***Have it dry:*** Greasy, fried foods are the rule rather than the exception at many restaurants. Butter and oil make foods taste better and, since taste is the primary concern of most chefs, they are used in abundance during cooking. However, this can add an enormous number of calories to a meal and clog your arteries with a profusion of unhealthy saturated fat. Realize that foods don't have to be greasy in order to be palatable. By using the right combination of spices, caloric balance can be maintained without sacrificing flavor. Hence, rather than opting for something fried, order your foods broiled, steamed, grilled or baked. To ensure that no additional fat is added, ask to have everything prepared "dry." And if the waiter gives you a hard time about this, just tell him that you're allergic to butter and oil. I guarantee he'll acquiesce and honor your request.

➡ ***Get it on the side:*** The secret of many recipes is in the sauce. Vodka, Alfredo and other cream-based mixtures help to give foods their distinct flavor. However, these condiments can turn an otherwise healthy meal into an all-out fat-fest (think filet of sole soaked in tartar sauce or salad greens smothered with bleu cheese dressing!). To keep calories in line, ask that any sauce or dressing be served on the side. Then, if you wish, lightly dip your food in the sauce—just enough to add some flavor. Remember: When it comes to sauce, less is more!

➡ ***Think brown:*** Rice, potatoes, bread and pasta are staples in restaurant fare. Although considered "complex" carbs, these foods tend to be high-glycemic in nature. Remember, high-glycemic foods are rapidly broken down into simple sugars, causing a spike in your blood-sugar levels. Consequently, your pancreas secretes large quantities of insulin as a means to clear the sugar from your bloodstream. Excess insulin is detrimental to weight management. It is directly responsible for converting sugars into body fat as well as inhibiting the conversion of stored fat into energy. This double-whammy greatly increases the potential for body-fat storage. Hence, rather than eating "white" starches, it is better to choose "brown" ones instead. For example, replace potatoes with yams, white rice with brown rice, refined pasta with the whole-wheat variety and plain bread with pumpernickel. These low-glycemic alternatives will keep blood sugar in check, helping to stabilize insulin secretions and thereby minimize fat storage.

➠ ***Eat your veggies:*** Your mother was right: Vegetables really are a nutritional panacea. Green vegetables, in particular, are an ideal food. They are replete in vitamins and minerals, devoid of saturated fat and extremely low in calories (a pound of broccoli, for example, contains only 120 calories). But there's an even more important reason why vegetables should be consumed: They suppress hunger. Because of their bulk, they take up a large amount of space in the stomach, helping to fill you up without filling you out. In effect, they are like green water—you can eat as much as you want without the fear of gaining weight. This is especially important in a restaurant setting, where the multitude of menu choices tend to encourage binge eating.

➠ ***Opt for fruit:*** Chocolate cheesecake, pie à la mode, tiramisu . . . there's no doubt that desserts tend to be the most fattening of all foods. The great majority are chock-full of sugar and saturated fat—a lethal combination in terms of promoting weight gain. Here is where you must exert a great deal of willpower. Passing up on sumptuous sweets requires the ability to forgo instant gratification for long-term benefit; not an easy task. Fruits are the perfect alternative. They are rich in fiber, plentiful in vitamins and minerals, and low on the glycemic scale (they don't cause a spike in insulin secretion). And, best of all, they taste great! Even if it's not on the dessert menu, a fruit plate can almost always be made to order; all you have to do is ask.

Putting It All Together

Table 10.1 summarizes the nutritional protocols that will help you look great sleeveless. Use these protocols as a guideline and adapt them to your individual needs. As previously stated, every woman is unique. Hence, there is no one best nutritional program. Experiment with different nutrient ratios and see how it affects your body. Over time, you'll find out what works best for you.

TABLE 10.1
NUTRITIONAL PROTOCOL

Nutrient	Recommended Percentage of Total Calories	Specific Recommendations
Carbohydrates	40 to 50%	• Eat low-glycemic carbs • Take in a high amount of fiber
Protein	30 to 40%	• Eat lean, high-quality protein sources
Fat	15 to 20%	• Eat mostly unsaturated, essential fatty acids

TIPS TO STAY LEAN

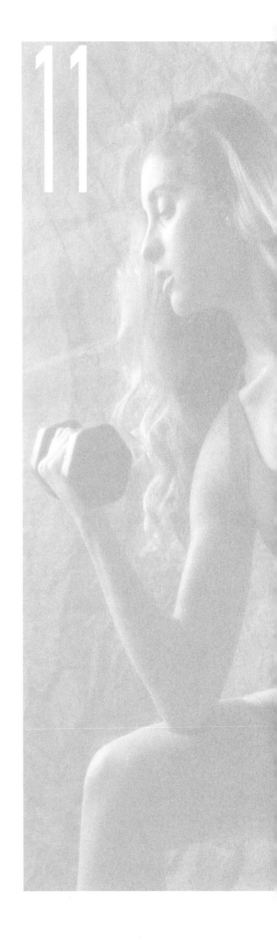

11

The complexities of nutrition go beyond carbs, protein and fat. While there's little doubt that the amount and proportion of these macronutrients are the dominant factors in weight management, other nutritional aspects can have a significant impact on your physique, too.

The following eight strategies will help to elevate your metabolism and maximize your body's fat-burning ability. By integrating these principles into your nutritional approach, it's possible to achieve a leaner physique without altering caloric intake. This is especially pertinent when it comes to shedding those last few pounds that always seem so hard to get rid of.

Eat Small, Frequent Meals

In today's fast-paced world, most women give little thought about the timing of their meals. All too often, breakfast consists only of a cup of coffee. Succeeding meals are eaten whenever there is a free moment, usually culminating with a large feast at dinner and possibly a midnight snack.

Unfortunately, this type of nutritional regimen has a deleterious effect on your body composition. When you deprive your body of food for more than a few hours, it senses that it won't have adequate fuel to carry out daily activities and shifts into a "starvation mode" as a means of conserving energy. Consequently, your metabolic rate slows down, preventing additional burning of calories. The end result is an increase in body-fat levels with a corresponding loss of lean muscle tissue.

By regimenting your eating patterns and consuming small, frequent meals, your body is able to operate at peak efficiency. Nutrients are better absorbed into your system, allowing them to be efficiently utilized for important biological functions. Your metabolism revs up, increasing your body's internal production of heat (a process called *thermogenesis*), which, in turn, helps to burn fat for fuel. Moreover, your appetite remains suppressed, making you less likely to binge out on a big meal late in the day.

There also is an expenditure of energy in the digestion process, called *dietary-induced thermogenesis*. Every time you eat, your body burns off approximately 10 percent of the calories consumed, keeping your metabolism elevated for up to several hours after consumption. By constantly taking in food, you increase dietary-induced thermogenesis and thus maintain a raised metabolic rate throughout the day.

Ideally, you should space out your meals evenly, eating five or six times a day at regular intervals. While this might seem like a time-consuming chore, it actually can be accomplished without a great deal of effort. For instance, you can prepare several meals in advance, store them in plastic containers, and reheat them in a microwave on an as-needed basis. As an alternative, you can supplement your basic meals with powdered meal replacements or sports bars. These "engineered foods" provide the ultimate in convenience: They are nutritionally balanced, easily transportable and can be prepared in a matter of minutes.

Decrease Starchy Carbs at Night

For most women, starchy carbs make up a substantial portion of their evening meals. Pasta, rice, potatoes . . . these are nightly staples in the standard American diet. Steak and fries, spaghetti and meatballs—what would dinner be without them?

The trouble with starchy carbs is that they are readily transformed to fat when eaten before bedtime. The reason for this is simple: The primary function of carbohydrates is to supply short-term energy for your daily activities. If carbs are not used immediately for fuel, they have two possible fates: They either are stored as glycogen in your liver and muscles or are converted into fatty acids and stored in adipose tissue as body fat. Since activity levels usually are lowest during the evening hours, there is a diminished use of carbs for fuel and therefore an increased potential for body-fat storage.

In general, the best time to consume carbs is early in the day, when your activity levels are at their peak. This will allow your body to utilize a maximal amount of carbs for energy and minimize the potential for fat deposition. Breakfast, in particular, is an excellent time to load up on complex carbs. A large bowl of rolled oats or bran cereal will set the stage for fueling your daily activities and keep you physically and mentally fit throughout the day.

On the other hand, it is best to limit your dinner fare to fibrous, vegetable-based carbohydrate sources. Fibrous vegetables tend to be extremely low in total calories and, because of their bulk, are very filling. For supper, consider eating a meal consisting of lean poultry or fish combined with a large bowl of salad greens. Other vegetables, such as broccoli, string beans, cauliflower and zucchini, also make fine nighttime carbohydrate choices and will reduce the potential for unwanted body-fat storage.

Stay Hydrated

Believe it or not, most of your body is made up of water. Your muscles are roughly 75-percent water, your blood is more than 80-percent water and your lungs are almost 90-percent water. Clearly, water is the most vital of all nutrients—without it, you would die in a matter of days.

Regrettably, some women cut back on their fluid intake, thinking that it will help to eliminate subcutaneous water retention. In some cases, they'll go so far as to refrain from drinking liquids altogether. What a big mistake! When fluids are restricted, your body senses a threat to its survival and tries to hold on to every last drop of water. The end result is an increase in water retention, leaving you puffy and bloated.

Worse, fluid restriction tends to make you fatter. Without an adequate supply of water, your kidney function becomes impaired, causing a systemic accumulation of metabolic waste. Your liver, in turn, has to work overtime to flush out these toxins from your body. This compromises your liver's ability to metabolize fat into usable energy—one of its primary responsibilities. As a result, less fat is metabolized, causing an increase in adipose storage.

In order to avoid this fate, water should be readily consumed. Aim to drink at least 3/4 of an ounce of fluids per pound of body weight, spacing out intake throughout the day. Alcohol- and caffeine-based beverages don't count toward this amount; they have a diuretic effect and actually cause you to dehydrate. Rather, your best bet is to drink plain old water, and a lot of it. Although tap water will suffice, natural spring water is a decidedly better choice. It is devoid of the pollutants that taint our reservoirs and therefore keeps your body free of contaminants. If possible, the water should be chilled or served on ice. Cold water is absorbed into the system more quickly than warm water, ensuring a continued state of hydration.

During exercise, fluid intake should be increased still further. As you work out, a large amount of water is lost through your sweat, breath and urine. If these fluids aren't replenished, your exercise performance is bound to suffer. In fact, a mere 3-percent reduction in water can cause up to a 10-percent loss in muscular strength. When taken to the extreme, heat stroke or even circulatory collapse can occur. Clearly, exercise-induced dehydration must be avoided at all costs.

It is a mistake, however, to rely on thirst as an indicator as to when to drink. Intense exercise inhibits the thirst sensors in your throat and gut; by the time you become thirsty, your body already is severely dehydrated. Therefore, during exercise, drink early and drink often. Consume 8 ounces of fluid immediately before your work-out and then take small sips of water every five or ten minutes or so while training.

Go Easy on the Sauce

The world floats on a sea of alcohol. Whether it's the two-martini lunch, the evening happy hour, or the after-dinner drink, alcohol is firmly ingrained in today's society. It is, without question, the most popular recreational drug in existence. In many circles, getting drunk even is a rite of passage—a rite that often continues throughout adulthood. With such widespread social acceptance, it's no wonder that approximately half of all Americans drink on a regular basis and more than 5 percent are heavy drinkers.

However, for any woman who aspires to maximize her body's potential, alcohol is a definite taboo. Make no mistake; alcohol will make you fat. It is calorically dense, containing over seven calories per gram (as opposed to carbs and protein, which have four). And this doesn't include the addition of mixers, which can significantly increase the calorie count. Take a look at the caloric content in some popular alcoholic beverages: A margarita has 600 calories; a martini, 250; and a beer, 150—pretty heavy stuff! What's more, these drinks are virtually devoid of any nutritional value. They are "empty calories" that do nothing but pack on unwanted pounds. Considering these facts, there is no doubt that even moderate drinking can have a decidedly negative impact on your figure.

Moreover, it is difficult for the body to break down alcohol. Your liver must use a tremendous amount of coenzymes (such as NAD and FAD) in order to assimilate the toxins from alcohol. Consequently, there are fewer coenzymes available to carry out vital metabolic functions (i.e., the Krebs cycle), including the breakdown of fat for energy. The end result: increased fat storage. This process can begin after just a single night of heavy drinking.

With chronic abuse, the consequences of alcohol can be disastrous—often irreparable. Alcohol is a poison. It infiltrates your internal organs and has a toxic effect on everything that it comes into contact with. Your liver and spleen, in particular, become severely impaired and lose their ability to carry out vital functions. Forget about losing body fat; your entire metabolic system becomes dysfunctional. And don't think your muscles are immune from the carnage. Sustained bouts of heavy drinking ultimately cause myopathy—a degeneration of muscle tissue that obliterates your hard-earned gains.

The best advice on alcohol is to limit consumption to an absolute minimum; if possible, eliminate it completely from your diet. Get used to the idea that you don't need alcohol to have a good time. If you're at a party or dance club, order a club soda with a twist of lemon or lime. Once you have adjusted to being a teetotaler, you'll soon appreciate the associated benefits. When others are in a drunken stupor, you'll be in full control of your faculties. You'll wake up hangover-free, never having to regret what you did the night before. And, of course, you'll keep your body operating at peak efficiency, maintaining optimal shape year-round.

Hold the Salt

Salt is the most widely used of all spices. It is added to almost every food imaginable, from soup to nuts and everything in between.

The craving for salt is physiologic. You see, there are distinct taste buds that are specifically receptive to salty foods. It is believed these taste buds reside on the tip and upper front portion of the tongue, producing a desire to consume salt.

Salt is comprised of sodium (as well as chloride), a basic mineral that's abundant in nature. Because it carries an electrical charge, sodium is considered an *electrolyte*. In conjunction with potassium, it is responsible for regulating the body's fluid balance; potassium maintains the fluid balance intracellularly (within the cells) while sodium maintains the balance of fluids extracellularly (outside the cells). Hence, sodium is essential for bodily function; a lack of it leads to hyponatremia, a condition that ultimately causes death.

Although it is an essential nutrient, only minute quantities of sodium are required through dietary means. In fact, a mere 500 milligrams is all that's needed to maintain normal biological function—an amount that equates to about 1/4 of a teaspoon of salt. Yet the average American consumes more than ten times this quantity! When too much sodium is ingested, fluid is drawn out of the cells and into the body's free spaces, causing the malady known as water retention. Your feet and hands swell, your face becomes puffy and water accumulates beneath your skin; not an enviable condition for someone trying to maintain a lean, toned physique. The fact is, sodium occurs naturally in most foods, and you'll get all you need just by eating a sensible diet.

The best way to avoid an overconsumption of sodium is by eating fresh, unprocessed foods. Stay away from all packaged and canned goods. They tend to be the worst offenders. Many condiments and sauces also are loaded with sodium.

Ketchup, salad dressings and soy sauce all contain whopping amounts. And in order to avoid any hidden sources, get used to reading food labels. The sodium content is plainly listed for all to see.

In addition, refrain from adding salt to your meals. If you want to spice up your foods, there are dozens of delicious seasonings that can enhance flavor without any side-effects. Paprika, cinnamon, basil, oregano, garlic—the list goes on. Experiment with different combinations and see what you find palatable. By using a little ingenuity, you can create tasty dishes that are virtually sodium-free.

Jumpstart with Java

Caffeine has gotten a bad rap. For years, health care practitioners have denounced it as a health hazard. They've cautioned against its use, citing studies that link it to everything from heart disease to cancer. However, the bulk of these studies were flawed in their design. Some used enormous quantities of caffeine—far beyond what the normal individual consumes. Others employed insufficient sample sizes or had errors in statistical analysis. The truth is, when all the available information is examined, there's really no evidence that modest caffeine consumption causes any detriments to overall health and well-being. In fact, a few studies actually found a negative correlation between caffeine and certain forms of cancer!

Does this mean that you should load up on caffeinated beverages? Absolutely not! Caffeine is a stimulant. At high doses, it can cause a host of unwanted side-effects such as hypertension, nervousness, insomnia and gastrointestinal distress. Guzzling massive quantities of coffee and cola will only serve to make you wired and irritable—not lean and defined.

However, when used in moderation, caffeine can be a safe and effective means of expediting a loss of body fat. By stimulating brown adipose tissue (BAT)—a special type of fat that elevates metabolism—caffeine facilitates the release of free fatty acids from adipocytes, allowing fat to be utilized for short-term energy. Studies have shown up to a 4-percent increase in resting metabolic rate from judicious caffeine supplementation, with effects lasting up to several hours after ingestion.

You don't need to take a lot of caffeine to derive positive benefits. A daily dose of 200 to 300 milligrams is all that's required to rev up your metabolic rate. Two cups of brewed coffee first thing in the morning will satisfy this requirement quite nicely. Better yet, consume the coffee immediately before your workout. In addition to its fat-burning effects, caffeine helps to delay fatigue and improve exercise intensity. Your performance will be enhanced, spurring you on to greater gains.

But remember to avoid going overboard with caffeine consumption. Excessive intake has no additional benefits and can actually impede results. When consumed in abundance, caffeine acts as a *vasoconstrictor*, narrowing arteries and restricting blood flow. As you may recall, a reduced circulatory capacity inhibits the breakdown of stored body fat. Ultimately, this counteracts the thermogenic effects of caffeine, nullifying its fat-burning benefits.

For best results, black coffee or espresso is recommended; the increased calories associated with adding cream or sugar will easily offset the caffeine-induced increase in metabolic rate. If black coffee is simply too bitter for your taste buds, then try using skim milk and/or artificial sweeteners as flavor enhancers.

An even better alternative to coffee is green tea. In addition to having caffeine, green tea contains special compounds called *catechin polyphenols* that increase the thermogenic effect of caffeine. Catechins inhibit an enzyme (called *catechol-O-methyl-transferase*) that degrades noradrenaline, a potent hormone that promotes the oxidation of body fat. In combination, caffeine and catechins act synergistically, enhancing resting energy expenditure beyond that of caffeine alone. Considering that it also is replete in vitamins and antioxidants (the benefits of which are discussed in the next section), green tea is a terrific beverage for keeping your body healthy and lean.

Have an Antioxidant Cocktail

Much has been made about vitamin and mineral supplementation. For many generations, these so-called micronutrients were touted as wonder supplements, heralded for curing everything from the common cold to night blindness. While we now know these claims to be greatly exaggerated, this doesn't diminish the fact that micronutrients are imperative for maintaining a fit, healthy body.

Vitamins and minerals serve many important biological functions. They facilitate energy transfer, prevent disease and act as coenzymes to assist in many chemical reactions. A deficiency in any of these micronutrients can lead to severe illness. Don't worry, though. If you follow the nutritional recommendations outlined in this book, you'll more than meet your daily requirements.

There is, however, a special class of micronutrients called *antioxidants,* which are required in much larger amounts than other vitamins and minerals. Antioxidants are the body's scavengers. They help to defend the body against damage caused by free radicals—unstable molecules that can injure healthy cells and tissues. Millions of these dangerous villains are produced each day during the normal course of respiration. The main culprit is oxygen. Every time you breathe, oxygen uptake causes free radical production. Environmental factors such as pollutants, smoke and certain chemicals also contribute to their formation. If left unchecked, free radicals can wreak havoc on your physique and cause a multitude of ailments, including arthritis, cardiovascular disease, dementia and cancer.

For the active woman, antioxidants are of particular importance. Due to increased oxygen consumption, free-radical production skyrockets during exercise. This results in an inflammation of muscle tissue, impairing muscular function and slowing recovery. The capacity for muscular repair is reduced, heightening the likelihood of overtraining.

Fortunately, like heroic warriors, antioxidants engulf free radicals, rendering them harmless. Not only does this improve your overall health and well-being, but it also improves your exercise capacity. There is a reduction in post-exercise muscle inflammation (with an associated decrease in delayed onset muscle soreness), helping to repair bodily tissues and speed recovery.

While there are dozens of known antioxidants, four of them are absolutely indispensable: vitamin C, vitamin E, coenzyme Q10 and alpha-lipoic acid. These antioxidants work synergistically with one another; their combined effect is greater than the sum of their individual actions. Other antioxidants that are beneficial include selenium, lycopene, isoflavones and polyphenols (although they don't have the synergistic capabilities of the "big four").

It is virtually impossible, however, to consume adequate quantities of antioxidants from food sources. For example, you'd have to drink eleven glasses of orange juice in order to get the recommended amount of vitamin C. Hence, supplementation is an absolute necessity. Table 11.1 lists the major antioxidants with corresponding dosages.

As a rule, it is best to consume supplements in conjunction with a meal. The absorption of micronutrients is improved when they are consumed with food. This also improves gastrointestinal tolerance of the supplement.

TABLE 11.1
RECOMMENDED DOSAGES OF ANTIOXIDANTS

Antioxidant	Dosage
Vitamin C	800 mg
Vitamin E	600 IU
Coenzyme Q10	50 mg
Alpha-lipoic acid	100 mg
Polyphenols	50 mg
Soy isoflavones	50 mg
Lycopene	10 mg
Selenium	200 mcg

IU = International Units.

Cheat a Little

Throughout the ages, food always has been a source of great temptation. Dating all the way back to Adam and Eve, there was the forbidden fruit; that luscious apple was simply too much to resist. Today, with food so plentiful, the temptations are literally endless. Let's face it, a great deal of willpower is required to pass up a slice of birthday cake or forego a bucket of chicken wings. For some, the thought of never again eating these types of foods is too much to bear. After several months of deprivation, they break down and go on an eating binge, scarfing down everything in sight.

To help keep your sanity, it is acceptable—even beneficial—to have a weekly "cheat" day. On your cheat day, you can eat basically anything you want, including sugar and/or fat-laden foods. Within reason, there are no restrictions. Go ahead and order a pizza. Frequent your favorite fast-food restaurant. Have a candy bar. Whatever your heart desires, feel free to indulge. You don't need to feel guilty about cheating; consider it a reward for sticking to your diet.

Try not to go too far overboard, though. While a little overindulgence won't have any effect on your physique, consuming mass quantities of food very well could (and it also can make you pretty sick!). Accordingly, don't allow the total calories on your cheat day to exceed more than 150 percent of your estimated daily intake. For instance, if you normally eat 1,600 calories, don't go past 2,400 calories. This will give you plenty of leeway to satisfy your food cravings while keeping caloric intake within a reasonable range.

Finally, make sure to limit cheating to no more than one day per week. Try to pick a specific cheat day and stay with it. Regimentation is an important part of maintaining a healthy lifestyle, and when cheating becomes a habit, regimentation goes by the wayside. Stick with the program and make your cheat day a special treat.

PREPARING FOR THE BIG EVENT

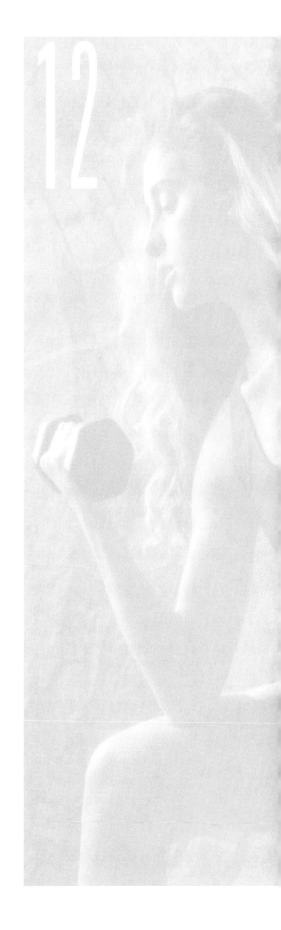

Okay, you've got it all together; you're training hard, eating right and living a fitness lifestyle. And your body is beginning to respond. You've lost inches off your waist and have started to see definition in places where you didn't even think you had muscles. All is going great, but you want more. You've got a big-time event coming up shortly and you really want to look your absolute best . . . .

Every so often, a specific occasion arises that drives a woman to pull out all the stops. It might be a wedding, a pool party, a high school reunion, or even a fitness or physique competition. You'll be in some sort of revealing outfit in front of a group of people, probably having to pose for an endless stream of photographs. Perhaps you'll be captured on video or, gasp, appear on TV!

If you are faced with such a situation, a specific nutritional regimen called carb depletion/carb loading is in order. The theory behind the strategy is simple. When carbs are drastically depleted, your body is forced to utilize all of its stored glycogen for energy.

Glycogen, if you remember, is the stored form of carbohydrate. It is abundant in the liver and muscles, providing a source of short-term energy. Why is this important? Well, glycogen is hydrophilic (it attracts water). For each gram of glycogen, the body stores approximately three grams of water.

Now here's where nutritional science comes in. By depleting glycogen, water is simultaneously excreted from your muscles and liver; the more glycogen you deplete, the more your body "dries out." Then, as soon as carbs are reintroduced, your muscles and liver rapidly take up glucose in order to replenish glycogen stores. More importantly, any water held subcutaneously (beneath the skin) is drawn into the cells along with the glycogen. If you do it right, your physique appears lean and hard, with full, shapely muscles that really stand out.

Realize, though, that a carb-depletion/carb-loading scheme is most effective when you are at or near your ideal body composition. It is not intended to be a quick-fix weight-loss program. Rather, it is a means to optimize your physique. If you are carrying a lot of body fat, the visible effects of the program will be seriously compromised.

Ideally, the diet should commence one week prior to the affair. For best results, adhere to the following protocols.

The Carb-Depletion Phase

Carb depletion should begin on the seventh day before the event and last for a total of three days. Hence, assuming the event is on a Saturday, carb depletion should begin on Sunday and last through Tuesday. The goal here is to dissipate all glycogen from your muscles and liver by the end of this phase.

The first step in the process is to drastically cut carbohydrate intake. A good rule of thumb is to limit carbs to no more than about 10 percent of total calories. The carbs that you do consume should be low-glycemic in nature and preferably contain some fiber to maintain regularity. It is advisable to ingest these carbs early in the day. Since glucose is the primary source of fuel for the brain and central nervous system, this will help to keep energy levels up. Oatmeal and whole wheat breads or cereals make excellent choices, as do unrefined grains. Green vegetables also are an important part of the mix and, since they are extremely low in caloric composition, can be consumed in abundance.

To make up for the reduction in carbs, approximately 50 percent of your calories should come from dietary fat. If desired, it's okay to eat foods high in saturated fat (such as bacon, hamburger and hard cheeses). Don't worry about any health consequences: the time frame is too short for intake of these products to have any negative effects on your well-being. Of course, mono and polyunsaturated sources (such as seeds, oils and nuts) are even better options and, if possible, should comprise the majority of fat consumption.

An excellent fat-based alternative is medium chain triglycerides (MCTs). MCTs are a special type of fat. They have a unique molecular structure that allows them to bypass the body's usual fat-storage mechanisms. Rather than breaking down into fatty acids, MCTs are transported directly into the liver where they are rapidly converted into an instant energy source. Due to this occurrence, the body prefers to utilize them for short-term fuel. So by including MCTs during carb depletion, you can help to maintain elevated energy levels without risking unwanted fat deposition. MCTs come in liquid form and can be added directly into foods and beverages. It can be purchased in most health food stores.

Protein should make up the balance of the diet, equating to roughly 40 percent of total calories. Although some people cut back on protein intake when carb depleting in order to minimize gluconeogenesis (the conversion of protein to glucose), this thinking is decidedly misguided. If protein intake is inadequate, the body is apt to cannibalize its muscle tissue for fuel—especially during times of caloric restriction. Only by keeping protein intake high will you attenuate any potential muscle loss. As far as gluconeogenesis, it's really a non-issue: The amount of protein conversion to glucose is relatively insignificant at this point and has little effect on glycogen resynthesis.

During the carb-depletion phase, you should work out every day, training all the major muscles of your body each time you exercise. Muscles lack an enzyme (called glucose-6-phosphatase) that allows glucose to be utilized in other bodily tissues. Since glucose is so important for muscular action, this is nature's way of preserving muscle glycogen for future use. Consequently, the only way to completely expend all of your muscle glycogen is by training the entire body.

As far as the mode of exercise, you can either choose to weight train or perform aerobics. If you decide to weight train, it's best to perform one exercise for each major muscle group. Very high reps (25 or more per set) are advisable, executing the movements in a slow, controlled fashion. It isn't necessary, though, to train with a great deal of intensity during this period. The concept is to facilitate glycogen depletion, not to develop your muscles. Consequently, you should terminate each set short of reaching muscular failure. One or two sets per muscle group will do the trick—any more and you risk overtraining.

If you prefer, light cardiovascular activity is an acceptable alternative to weight training. Again, make sure to utilize exercises that work the entire body. The treadmill or bike alone simply won't do. You also need to incorporate an upper body aerobic movement such as rowing, elliptical training or cross-country skiing. Keep intensity relatively low, staying in a range of about 60 to 70 percent of maximal heart rate.

It's important to realize that by the end of the three-day depletion phase, your body won't look like you want it to. Your muscles will be flat and your face will be drawn. What's more, you'll probably feel a little weak and lethargic. Don't worry! Once you carb load, all of these effects will be reversed. Provided you stick with the protocols, all will be well by that special day.

Table 12.1 lists the protocols for the carb-depletion phase.

TABLE 12.1

PROTOCOLS FOR THE CARB-DEPLETION PHASE

Nutrient	Percentage of Total Calories
Carbohydrate	10
Protein	40
Fat	50

The Carb-Loading Phase

Carb loading should begin four days out and last for two more days. So for the same Saturday event, carb loading will take place on Wednesday and Thursday. You now want to replenish all of your glycogen stores, achieving a phenomenon known as glycogen supercompensation.

During this phase, jack up carbohydrate intake to around 60 percent of total calories. Consume mostly low-glycemic carbs such as brown rice, yams, oatmeal and other whole grains. Vegetables should be kept to a minimum, as they will fill you up without doing much to enhance glycogen uptake. To ensure maximal absorption, spread out carb intake throughout the day, eating small amounts with every meal.

Dietary fat—particularly of the saturated variety—must be avoided at all costs. Due to the high carbohydrate consumption, insulin levels will be consistently elevated during this phase. If you remember, insulin is a storage hormone and turns on various mechanisms that promote the deposition of body fat. Hence, when excess fats are consumed in conjunction with high levels of insulin, the potential for fat storage is significantly increased. You therefore should consume only essential fatty acids (such as flaxseed or fish oil) and keep intake to about 10 percent of calories.

Protein will make up the balance of calories (approximately 30 percent of total caloric intake). As opposed to the depletion phase, you now must stay clear of bacon, cheeses and creams since they are extremely high in fat. Stick with lean protein sources such as white meat poultry, egg whites and protein powders.

You should refrain from performing any type of exercise during this period. While you might be inclined to believe that training right up until the end is beneficial, it's not. In fact, it's actually counterproductive. Working out only serves to deplete the very glycogen stores that you're trying to replenish. You'll end up looking flat and stringy—not full and hard. Hence, resist any temptation to go to the gym, regardless of the psychological urge to train.

You can, however, perform isotension (described in Chapter 3) during carb loading. If you are preparing for a physique-oriented competition, this technique is especially beneficial. It will help to increase your muscular endurance and allow you to hold your poses for extended periods of time. Sessions can be expanded to 20 minutes or so, posing each of the body's major muscle groups.

Table 12.2 lists the protocols for the carb-loading phase.

TABLE 12.2

PROTOCOLS FOR THE CARB-LOADING PHASE

Nutrient	Percentage of Total Calories
Carbohydrate	60
Protein	30
Fat	10

Final Preparation

Finally, on the last day before the event, carb intake should be adjusted based on your appearance—increasing them if you look flat or reducing them if you appear bloated. Assuming you've nailed it on the head, you should be right on for your special occasion!

On the "big day" you should again assess your physique. While your ability to significantly change your appearance is limited at this point, minor adjustments can still be made. If all is well, stick with small portions of dried fruit right up until the time of the event.

A final note: People respond differently to a carb-deplete/carb-load scheme. It is therefore beneficial to experiment with this technique several months before your event. This is particularly important if you are entering a physique-oriented competition. If you're going to be judged on your appearance in comparison with other women, you certainly don't want to tempt fate. Once you go through the regimen once or twice, you'll be comfortable with how your body reacts and you'll be able to make adjustments based on your individual response.

RECIPES OF THE TOP FITNESS MODELS

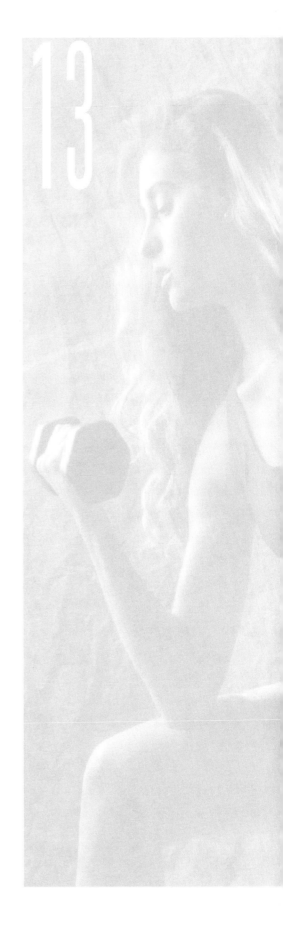

You really can eat healthy foods that actually taste great!
Just because a dish is low in fat and sugar doesn't mean
that it has to be bland.

I asked some of the top fitness models in the
world—women who make their living by looking
great—to submit their favorite healthy recipes. Here are
their mouth-watering responses. You'll find everything
from breakfast, lunch and dinner entrées, to snacks.
And, best of all, most of the recipes take only minutes
to prepare.

So go ahead and indulge yourself. Eat like a champion and enjoy!

TINA JO ORBAN
Professional Swimsuit Model
www.tinajoorban.com

TINA JO'S
LOW-CAL SQUASH AND APPLE SOUP

Ingredients:

1½ cups water

2 medium large Golden Delicious apples

2 medium butternut squash

2 tbsp. extra-virgin olive oil

1 small chopped onion

1 can vegetable broth

1 tbsp. chopped fresh thyme

1 tsp. salt

⅛ tsp. course ground pepper

1 cup one-percent low-fat milk

Directions:

Peel and core each apple and cut into ¾-inch chunks. With large chef's knife, cut squash into 2 pieces and slice off the peel. Remove and discard seeds. Cut squash into small ½-inch pieces. In large saucepan, heat oil on medium heat, add onion and cook until tender. Stir in apples, squash, broth, thyme, salt, pepper and water; heat to boil on high. Reduce heat to low; cover and simmer, stirring frequently for about 20 to 25 minutes or until squash is tender. Spoon ⅓ of mixture into a blender. Cover and blend at low speed until smooth. Pour mixture into bowl. Repeat with remaining mixture. Return the blended mixture to saucepan, stir in milk and heat over medium heat, stirring occasionally; DO NOT BOIL. Pour into your favorite large soup bowl, garnish with fresh chopped thyme and enjoy!

THERESA HESSLER

Jan Tana Pro Fitness Classic Champion
www.theresahessler.com

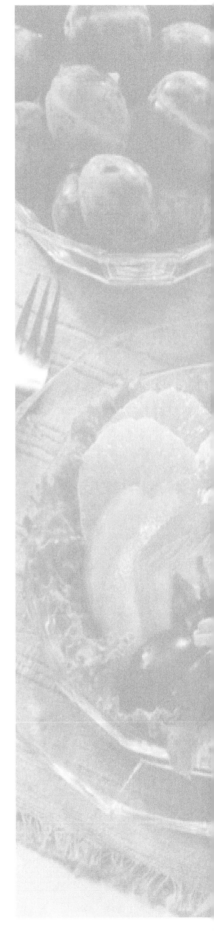

THERESA'S TURKEY CUTLETS

Ingredients:

Package of turkey breast cutlets or turkey tenderloins, halved

½ tbsp. olive oil

Italian bread crumbs

1 whole egg

2 tbsps low-fat mozzarella cheese

1 jar tomato sauce of your choice

Directions:

Heat olive oil in a fry pan (use just enough to coat bottom of pan). Dip turkey breasts in egg and coat with Italian bread crumbs. Place in fry pan and brown each side of cutlet. Place cutlet in a glass baking dish and spread tomato sauce over the top of cutlets. Cook for 20 minutes at 350°. During the last 5 minutes, sprinkle cheese over the top of cutlets. Serve hot and enjoy!

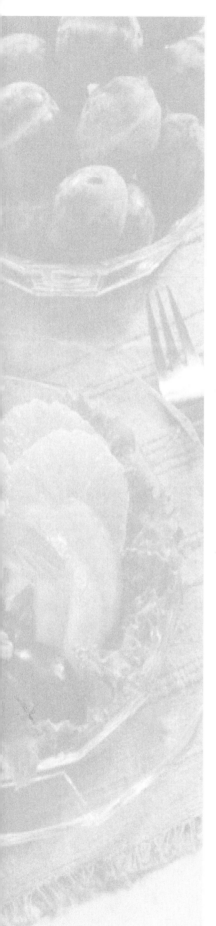

KAREN HULSE

Ms. World Professional Fitness Champion
Centrex Sports Club
887 Rt. 35 N.
Middletown, NJ 07748
www.karenhulse.com

KAREN'S
LEAN CHILI

Ingredients:

2 lbs. 93-percent lean ground beef
1 large can tomato puree
2 cans red kidney beans
2 packages chili seasoning
Optional: low-fat or fat-free shredded cheddar cheese

Directions:

In a large skillet or stir-fry pan, brown ground beef and drain excess fat. Add kidney beans, tomato puree and chili seasoning. Cook for 10 minutes, top with cheese, and enjoy!

CYNTHIA HILL

Ms. Galaxy
www.cynthiahill.com
(714) 294-2257

CYNTHIA'S
PROTEIN OATMEAL COOKIES

Ingredients:

5 egg whites

1 whole egg

½ cup fat-free spread

½ cup pure cane golden brown sugar

3 packets artificial sweetener

1 tsp. vanilla

1 cup vanilla protein powder

½ cup all-purpose flour

1 tsp. baking soda

½ tsp. salt

4 cups oats

Directions:

Heat oven to 350°. Beat together fat-free spread and sugars until creamy. Add eggs and vanilla, beat well; add combined flour, protein powder and baking soda, and mix well. Stir in oats and mix all ingredients together; drop by rounded heaping tablespoonfuls onto ungreased cookie sheet. Bake 12–15 minutes or until golden brown. Enjoy!

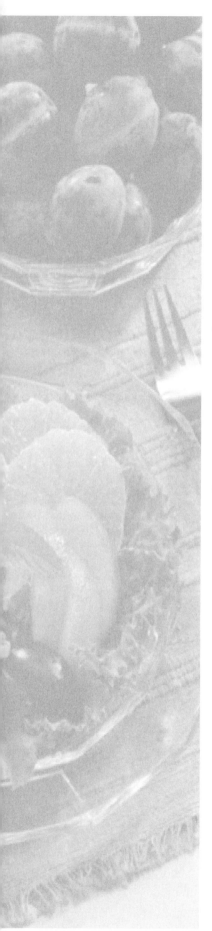

NICOLE ROLLOLAZO

Fitness America Champion 2000

www.nicolefitness.com

NICOLE'S LEAN TURKEY SALAD

Ingredients:

Mixed greens
Cilantro
Lean ground turkey breast
Fat-free Parmesan cheese
Lemon juice and pepper

Directions:

Cook the ground turkey until lightly browned. Add fresh cilantro into the mixed green salad, then sprinkle the turkey, cheese, pepper and lemon juice over the top. Toss and enjoy!

JEN HENDERSHOTT

NPC USA Fitness Champion
E-mail: jenhenfit2000@aol.com
Voice mail: (614) 520-3510
www.jennyh.com

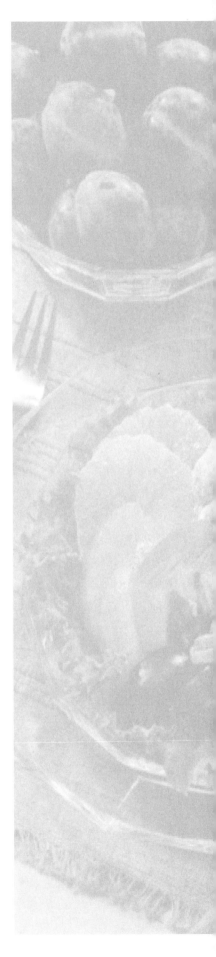

JEN'S
HEALTHY THIN-CRUST PIZZA

Ingredients:

1 thin pizza crust

Several tablespoons barbecue sauce (to taste)

1 chicken breast, cut into cubes

Several tablespoons fat-free shredded Parmesan cheese
(to taste)

Directions:

Grill chicken breast cubes until lightly browned. Spread barbecue sauce evenly over pizza crust. Sprinkle Parmesan cheese over the barbecue sauce. Place chicken cubes in select areas over top. Bake for 10–15 minutes. Serve hot and enjoy!

NANCY GEORGES

Ms. Fitness USA

www.nancygeorges.com

NANCY'S
SPICY SALSA TURKEY

Ingredients:

4 ounces instant rice

5 ounces ground lean turkey breast

2 tsp. chili powder

3 heaping tsp. medium salsa

Directions:

Sprinkle chili powder over turkey and grill until brown. Simultaneously boil rice until moist. Combine turkey and rice in large bowl and add salsa. Mix together and enjoy!

SUSAN BALSON

Hawaiian Tropic Ms. Fit California

www.fitbeauty.com

SUSAN'S "MOCK" BEEF STROGANOFF

Ingredients:

1 lb. 96-percent lean ground beef

1 12 oz. package pasta of your choice

1 can 98-percent fat-free mushroom soup

8 ounces fat-free sour cream

1 package onion soup

Directions:

Fill medium pot with hot water. Set pot on stove on high heat. While waiting for pasta water to boil, brown ground beef in large skillet, making sure to keep ground beef in as small pieces as possible. Empty ground beef into colander and then rinse with scalding hot water for 30 seconds (this flushes out some cooked unnecessary fat), then briskly wash skillet. Set aside. Add pasta to boiling water. Add ground beef to skillet; while simmering, add soup packet, stirring for 1–2 minutes. Add mushroom soup and fat-free sour cream. Stir until well blended, continuing to simmer for 2–4 minutes, allowing flavors to meld. Cook pasta till al denté, drain, then toss into skillet mixture and enjoy!

CONNIE GARNER

Ms. World Fitness
P.O. Box 1755
Queanbeyan NSW 2620
Australia
www.connieg.com

CONNIE'S
TUNA MARINARA

Ingredients:

1 medium can tuna in spring water
1 can chopped tomatoes
1 tub low-fat cottage cheese
1 small onion (or spring onion), chopped
Herbs and spices of your choice

Directions:

In a fry pan or saucepan (without oil or butter), dry fry the onions. Add the tuna and cook for about one minute; add herbs, spices and tomatoes, and simmer for about three minutes. Add the cottage cheese and simmer for another two minutes. Serve hot and enjoy!

TATIANA ANDERSON

Ms. Fitness USA

www.tatianaanderson.com

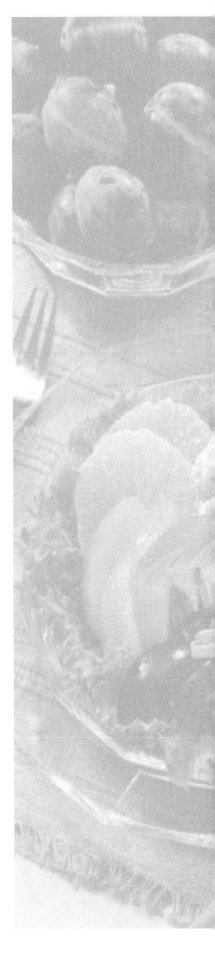

TATIANA'S CINNAMON FRITTATA

Ingredients:

Non-stick cooking spray

½ cup cooked cream of rice

6 egg whites

¼ tsp. vanilla extract

¼ tsp. almond extract

¼ tsp. Molly McButter™

¼ tsp. cinnamon

3 packets artificial sweetener

Directions:

Preheat 6-inch Teflon® pan, that has been sprayed with non-stick cooking spray, over medium heat. Mix cream of rice, extracts and sweetener together. Fold into egg whites and mix well. Pour mixture into pan and cover. Cook for 5 to 10 minutes (until solid), turn over, and sprinkle with Molly McButter™ and cinnamon. Cook one more minute and enjoy!

TANJA BAUMANN
Miss Fitness Switzerland
www.tanja-baumann.ch/

TANJA'S
SWISS-STYLE MUESLI

Ingredients:

14 ounces muesli mix (oat flakes, raisins, sunflower seeds,
nuts and cornflakes)

1 pint skim milk

8 ounces low-fat yogurt

8 ounces low-fat fromage frais (curd cheese)

1 large grated apple

2 medium bananas

2 tsp. honey

Directions:

Gently hand-stir the ingredients, while slowly adding the milk
for texture. Wait 5 to 10 minutes to let the mixture set. Fill 6
to 8 bowls and enjoy!

KIM KANNER

Professional Wrestling Valet

www.Kim Kanner.com

Kim's Grilled Shrimp Wraps

Ingredients:

Non-stick cooking spray

1 lb. shrimp

⅓ cup reduced-fat unsalted peanut butter

¼ cup honey

3 tbsps. soybean paste

2 tbsps. water

2 tbsps. fresh lime juice

12 romaine lettuce leaves

2 cups julienne-cut carrots

2 cups julienne-cut jicama

1 cup julienne-cut seedless cucumber

1 cup fresh bean sprouts

1 cup shredded red cabbage

Directions:

Grill shrimp using non-stick cooking spray on a skillet. Combine peanut butter, honey, soybean paste, water and lime juice in a bowl with a whisk and set aside. Cut the raised portion or vein off each romaine lettuce leaf (this will make the leaf more pliable to roll as a wrap). Combine the remaining ingredients and divide grilled shrimp into equal portions on lettuce leaves and roll. Then secure each wrap with a toothpick. Serve with sauce drizzled on top and enjoy!

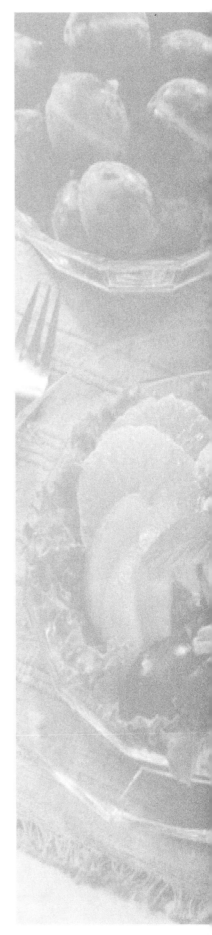

SHANNON METERAUD

Ms. Super Fitness
c/o JMP Management
P.O. Box 293
Presto, PA 15142
www.jmpmanagement.com

SHANNON'S
SWEET AND TANGY STEAK

Ingredients:

Non-stick cooking spray
7-oz. flank steak (sliced very thin)
3 packets artificial sweetener
Mustard to taste
Brown rice

Directions:

Place thinly sliced flank steak in a bowl. Add artificial sweetener. Add mustard according to taste. Mix together with a fork until the steak is covered. Place in a skillet sprayed with non-stick cooking spray. Cook until steak is a little brown (I like mine a little crispy). Serve with brown rice and enjoy!

CIE ALLMAN

Television Fitness Personality

www.vitamincie.com

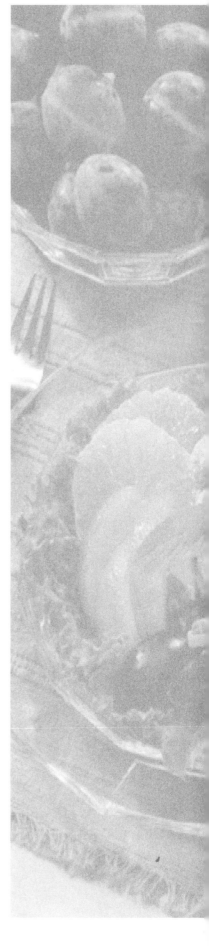

CIE'S
RASPBERRY CHICKEN AND
GOAT-CHEESE SALAD

Ingredients:

8 ounces chicken breast

½ head romaine lettuce

Fat-free raspberry and balsamic dressing (to taste)

1 tbsp. goat cheese

Directions:

On a gas or electric burner, preheat a non-stick pan at 400°. Cut up chicken into bite-sized pieces or strips and cook until brown. Place chicken on a bed of lettuce and sprinkle goat cheese over the top. Add the raspberry dressing and enjoy!

Appendix A
HIGH-FIBER FOODS

FOOD	AMOUNT	FIBER CONTENT (G)
Apple	Medium	3
All-Bran® cereal	1 ounce	10
Barley	1 cup	6
Black beans	1 cup	19
Blackberries	1 cup	8
Bread (whole wheat)	2 slices	6
Broccoli	1 cup	8
Chick peas	1 cup	12
Corn	Medium ear	5
Green peas	1 cup	18
Lentils	1 cup	15
Oatmeal	½ cup	4
Pear	Medium	4
Raspberries	1 cup	9
Rice (brown)	½ cup	5
Spinach	1 cup	7
Yams	Medium	7

GLOSSARY OF TERMS

Adipocyte. Fat cell.

Aerobic Exercise. Any activity that allows your body to consistently replenish oxygen to your working muscles. It is performed at a low to moderate intensity and is endurance-oriented by nature. Both fat and glycogen are burned for fuel.

Alpha-2 Receptor. "Entrance" that allows fat to enter an adipocyte.

Anaerobic Exercise. Any activity that utilizes oxygen at a faster rate than your body can replenish it in the working muscles. By nature, this type of exercise is intense and short in duration. Glycogen is the primary source of fuel.

Barbell. A long bar, usually measuring about six feet in length, that can accommodate weighted plates on each end. The Olympic barbell is the industry standard and weighs 45 pounds.

Bench. An apparatus designed for performing exercises in a seated or lying fashion. Many benches are adjustable so that exercises can be performed at a wide array of different angles.

Beta Receptor. "Exit" that allows fat to escape an adipocyte.

Bodysculpting. The art of shaping your muscles to optimal proportions.

Cardio. Short for cardiovascular (aerobic) exercise.

Circuit Training. A series of exercise machines set up in sequence. The exercises are performed one after the other, each stressing a different muscle group.

Collar. A clamp that secures weighted plates on a barbell or dumbbell.

Compound Movement. An exercise that involves two or more joints in the performance of the movement. Examples include squats, bench presses and chins.

Contraction. The act of shortening a muscle.

Cross Training. Using two or more different exercises in a routine. Generally used in the context of aerobic activities.

Definition. The absence of fat in the presence of well-developed muscle.

Dumbbell. A shortened version of a barbell, usually measuring about 12 inches in length, that allows an exercise to be performed one arm at a time.

Estrogen. Primary female hormone. Linked to increased fat storage.

Exercise. An individual movement that is intended to tax muscular function.

Failure. The point in an exercise where you cannot physically perform another rep.

Flexibility. A litheness of the joints, muscle and connective tissue that dictates range of motion.

Form. The technique utilized in performing the biomechanics of an exercise.

Free Weights. Barbells and dumbbells. These are opposed to exercise machines.

Giant Set. A series of three or more exercises performed in succession without any rest between sets.

Hypertrophy. An increase in muscle mass.

Intensity. The amount of effort involved in a set.

Isolation Movement. An exercise that involves only one joint in the performance of the movement. Examples include cable crossovers, biceps curls and leg extensions.

Nautilus™. A brand of exercise equipment found in many health clubs. The term has become synonymous with any exercise machine.

Plates. Flat, round weights that can be placed at the end of a barbell or dumbbell.

Progesterone. Primary female hormone. Linked to increased appetite.

Pump. The pooling of blood in a muscle due to intense anaerobic exercise.

Repetition (Rep). One complete movement of an exercise.

Resistance. The amount of weight used in an exercise.

Rest Interval. The amount of time taken between sets.

Routine. The configuration of exercises, sets and reps that you utilize in a training session.

Set. A series of repetitions performed in succession.

Symmetry. The way in which muscle groups complement one another, creating a proportional physique.

Testosterone. Primary male hormone. Responsible for promoting muscle mass.

Thermogenesis. Increased body heat. Accelerates fat burning.

INDEX

ABOUT THE AUTHOR

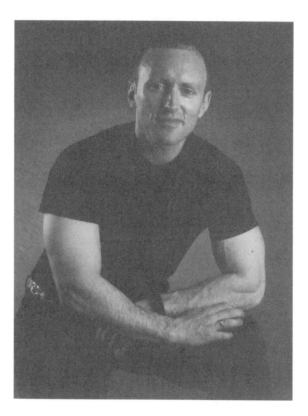

Brad Schoenfeld is widely regarded as one of America's leading fitness experts. He is the author of the best-selling fitness books *Sculpting Her Body Perfect* and *Look Great Naked*. He has been published or featured in virtually every major magazine (including *Cosmopolitan, Self, Marie Claire, Fitness, Shape,* and dozens of others) as well as appearing on hundreds of television shows and radio programs across the United States. Certified as a strength and conditioning specialist (by the National Strength and Conditioning Association) and as a personal trainer (by both the American Council on Exercise and Aerobics and Fitness Association of America), he was awarded the distinction of being classified as a Master Trainer by the International Association of Fitness Professionals. A frequent lecturer on both the professional and consumer level, Schoenfeld lives in Croton-on-Hudson, New York.